BIOMEDICAL ENGINEERING

A. EDWARD PROFIO, Ph.D.
Professor of Biomedical Engineering
University of California, Santa Barbara

JOHN WILEY & SONS, INC.

New York / Chichester / Brisbane / Toronto / Singapore

Library of Congress Cataloging in Publication Data:
Profio, A. Edward, 1931–
    Biomedical engineering / A. Edward Profio.
        p.   cm.
    Includes bibliographical references.
    ISBN 0-471-57768-5 :
    1. Biomedical engineering.   I. Title.

    R856.P76   1993
    610' .28—dc20   92-27830
                                                         CIP

Printed in the United States of America

10 9 8 7 6 5 4 3 2

Dedicated to my grandchildren

TABLE OF CONTENTS

PREFACE

This book is intended for juniors, seniors, and graduate students in engineering, and for researchers. It covers the application of engineering principles to medicine, with special emphasis on diagnostic and therapeutic instrumentation. Mechanical and mathematical models of physiology are also discussed. Because most engineers have little if any acquaintance with biology, a brief survey of human anatomy and physiology is included. The book also discusses sensors (transducers) and applications to physiological measurements, as well as systems using various sensors and effectors for diagnosis, therapy, or rehabilitation. Materials compatible with body tissues and blood are treated. Diagnostic devices based on light, x-rays, gamma rays from radioisotopes, ultrasound, and magnetic fields are discussed. The therapeutic devices included are basically artificial organs, lasers, and x-rays from electron accelerators.

Engineers have made great contributions to medical diagnosis and therapy. For example, the technique of computed tomography (CT) was developed by engineers. Engineers are intimately involved in laser surgery and other laser applications. However, a medical doctor must use the instruments and develop the best method of applying them without harm to the patient. A team consisting of a biomedical engineer and a physician or surgeon is involved in most new developments, and communication between them must be cultivated because of their widely differing education and experience. This goes beyond the matter of terminology. The physician seldom has a background in research and is unfamiliar with advanced physics and mathematics. The engineer lacks detailed knowledge of the human body and disease, and is not trained or licensed to treat patients. Therefore, this book provides a guide to medical terminology and use of instruments in medical practice.

Ethical standards and governmental regulations on human experimentation must be followed. A local committee usually reviews the proposed research. The patient must give informed consent to the procedure, and subjects whose free consent may be questionable (those of limited intelligence, those with mental illness, and prisoners) must not be used. An example of informed consent is included in Appendix C.

The biomedical engineer may use cells, tissues, animals for at least the initial experiments and tests of a new technique. There are many regulations on animal research, aimed at making sure the animals are treated humanely and that unnecessary numbers of them are not used. There must usually be a veterinarian on the staff, as well as a committee to review research proposals for appropriateness and compliance with governmental regulations and ethical standards. Animals cannot substitute for humans in all situations, but mammals such as mice, rats, rabbits, and hamsters are widely used. For experiments involving brain function, a monkey or another primate may be substituted. Safety precautions are important, especially to prevent transmission of disease. Animal experimentation is discussed in Appendix B.

I wish to acknowledge my wife and children, Janet, Christopher, Claudia, and Susan, who have been patient throughout the writing and revision of this book, the students in my biomedical engineering class who have inspired this work, faculty members and others who have contributed their expertise, and my medical colleagues over the years.

A. Edward Profio

Santa Barbara, California

CHAPTER 1

INTRODUCTION

1.0 SCOPE OF BIOMEDICAL ENGINEERING

Biomedical engineering has been defined as the application of principles of engineering, mathematics, and physical science to problems in biology and medicine. Such a problem is usually related to (1) the modeling of normal or abnormal human physiology or (2) research and design of instrumentation and machines for medical diagnosis or therapy. Thus the field might also be termed *medical engineering. Clinical engineering* might be used to identify work done within a hospital or other clinical setting.

Biomedical or medical engineering is closely allied to medical physics. One might consider medical physics to be a part of biomedical engineering. Historically, the medical physicist has concentrated on radiological physics, especially radiotherapy. Medical physics now encompasses other diagnostic and therapeutic modalities as well. The only real distinction is that a medical physicist has a degree in physics rather than in engineering.

Biophysics and *bioengineering* are broader terms, involving almost any interaction of physics or engineering with biology or medicine. Biophysicists, for example, may investigate fundamental physicochemical properties of biomembranes. A biochemical engineer uses cells or organisms to produce chemicals. A biotechnologist ("genetic engineer") may create new organisms using recombinant DNA techniques.

The biomedical engineer is a professional-level engineer and must not be confused with a technician or technologist, who may operate and maintain apparatus but not carry out original research or design. Nevertheless, a biomedical engineer should know how to operate equipment and must be concerned with other pertinent matters, such as laboratory safety, discussed in Appendix A. The concept of a professional engineer in this field is often unfamiliar to medical doctors, and biomedical engineers are sometimes called medical physicists instead. In any case, it is important for these professionals to develop a good working relationship with a physician or surgeon if clinical work is to be performed, because neither an engineer nor a physicist is educated or licensed to diagnose or treat patients.

A well-educated biomedical engineer should know something of biology and medicine, and the more the better. He or she should also be educated in an engineering discipline (or in physics). The discipline may be biomedical engineering, electrical engineering, chemical engineering, computer science or engineering, materials science or engineering, mechanical engineering, or nuclear engineering. Departments of biomedical engineering usually emphasize one or more aspects of the other fields, depending on faculty interests, but give the broadest education. Electrical engineering typically covers electronic sensors for physiological monitoring, analysis of ECG (electrocardiogram) and EEG (electroencephalogram) signals, and other applications. Chemical engineering may involve chemical sensors and control, kidney dialysis machines, and related subjects. Computer science is often applied to digital image processing and other applications of computers to medicine. Materials engineering may include biomaterials compatible with tissues. Mechanical engineering may involve modeling blood flow, designing artificial organs, and so forth. Nuclear engineering is related to radiological physics (radiotherapy, diagnostic x-rays, and nuclear medicine).

Career opportunities exist in medical institutions, medical equipment and service companies, universities, and government or private research institutes. Recent advances in medical technology, such as computed tomography (CT) and nuclear magnetic resonance imaging (MRI), suggest the possibilities for future breakthroughs and indicate an increased demand for biomedical engineers.

1.1 TERMINOLOGY

One of the greatest impediments to communication between engineers and medical personnel is, on one hand, medical terminology and, on the other, engineering terminology and mathematical expressions. It is important for the biomedical engineer to learn essential medical terminology.

There are innumerable anatomical terms, but they do not have to be learned all at once. One can concentrate on the part of the body or system of current concern. Anatomy can be learned from various texts and reference books (for example, those listed in the Bibliography that follows each chapter in this book) or, even better, in the laboratory.

Some useful terms describing anatomical location and direction are shown in Fig. 1.1. Note that the body is in the standard anatomical position: standing, with the arms at the sides and the palms of the hands facing forward. The

a median plane
b sagittal plane
c frontal plane
d transverse plane
e cranial direction
f caudal direction
g anterior
h posterior
i medial
j lateral
k proximal
l distal

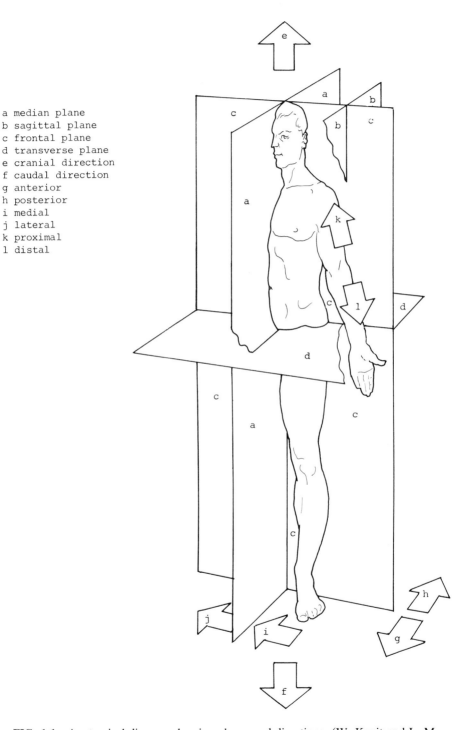

FIG. 1.1   Anatomical diagram showing planes and directions. (W. Kapit and L. M. Elson, Anatomy Coloring Book, Harper & Row, New York, 1977)

TABLE 1.1   Medical Terms

Prefixes

a-, an-, ar-	without, not lack of	ab-, ad-	away from, toward
leuco-	white	ante-, pre-	before
brachy-	near	brady-	slow
dia-, trans-	through	dys-	bad, painful
ecto-	outside	endo-	within
epi-	upon	eu-	good
hyper-	over	hypo-	under
infra-	below	inter-	between
intra-	within	macro-	large
micro-	small	ortho-	straight
para-	near, beside	pseudo-	false
postero-	behind	sclero-	hard
super-	above	tachy-	rapid
xero-	dry		

Suffixes

-algia	pain	-centesis	surgical puncture
-ectasis	dilation, expansion	-ectomy	excision, removal
-emia	blood	-gen	producing
-gram	record	-graph	recording instrument
-graphy	process of recording	-iasis, -osis	abnormal condition
-itis	inflammation	-lysis	dissolution
-megaly	enlargement	-meter	measuring instrument
-oma	tumor	-plasty	plastic repair
-otomy	incision	-pathy	disease
-penia	deficiency	-rrhage	burst forth, bleed
-rrhea	discharge, flow	-scopy	examination, view
-spasm	involuntary, contraction	-tripsy	crush

Word Root (combining form)

aden	gland	adip, lip	fat
angi, vas	vessel	arteri	artery
arthr	joint	ather	fatty deposit
cardi	heart	cephal	head
cervic	neck	chol	bile
chondr	cartilage	cost	rib
crani	skull	cutane, derm	skin
cyst	bladder	cyt	cell
gastr	stomach	hem	blood
hepat	liver	hist	tissue
mamma, mast	breast	morph	shape
my	muscle	myel	bone marrow, spinal cord
nephr, ren	kidney	oste	bone
phleb, ven	vein	pulmon	lung
splen	spleen or diaphragm	squam	scale
stasis	not moving	stoma	stomach
thorac	chest	thromb	clot
vertebr	vertebra		

median plane divides the body into left and right halves. A *sagittal plane* divides the body into unequal left and right parts and is parallel to the median plane. The terms *medial* and *lateral* refer to this plane. The *coronal* or *frontal plane* divides the body into equal or unequal front and back parts. The terms *anterior* and *posterior* refer to this plane. The *horizontal plane* divides the body into upper (cranial) and lower (caudal) parts. *Cross* or *transverse planes* are perpendicular to the long axis of the body. *Cranial* or *superior* refers to a structure that is closer to the head, or higher, than another structure. *Caudal* or *inferior* refers to a structure that is closer to the feet, or lower, than another structure. *Anterior* or *ventral* refers to a structure that is more to the front than another structure. *Posterior* or *dorsal* refers to a structure that is more to the back than another structure. *Medial* means closer to the median plane, whereas *lateral* means farther away from the median plane. *Proximal* means closer to the root of a limb (or median plane) or to another reference point. *Distal* means farther from the root of a limb (or median plane) or to another reference point.

A few common medical terms are listed in Table 1.1. Medical terms are usually derived from Latin or Greek. Medical words are often compound, consisting of the combining form of a wood root and a prefix, a suffix, or both. The prefix or suffix is often linked by *o* if the following part begins with a consonant. For example, xeroradiography is a dry (*xero*) process using x-ray radiation (*radio*) for producing an image or record (*graph*). Sometimes both Latin and Greek roots are used. For instance, the Latin word for breast is *mamma*, whereas the Greek word is *mastos*; thus, *mammography* (referring to an to x-ray of the breast), but *mastectomy* (surgical excision of the breast). Other terms can be found in the references on medical terminology listed in the Bibliographies and in medical dictionaries, which also give the pronunciation.

1.2   MEASUREMENTS AND STATISTICS

Biomedical engineering, like other branches of engineering and science, is characterized by quantitative measurements. Measurements of physical quantities are subject to errors, which are of two kinds; systematic, and random (or statistical). The *accuracy* of a measurement relates to the closeness of the *mean* to the true value. Because the true value is usually unknown, accuracy is evaluated by comparison of the measured mean of the observations to a standard. Ideally, this is a standard traceable to the primary standard for that quantity maintained at the National Institute of Science and Technology. In practice, one usually *calibrates* the apparatus to ensure adequate accuracy for the measurement. *Precision* refers to the statistical variation of a measurement from the mean. It is usually expressed in terms of plus or minus the standard deviation, which is discussed later.

Figure 1.2 shows a typical static calibration curve for a transducer (a device that senses one form of energy, or other quantity, and transforms it into

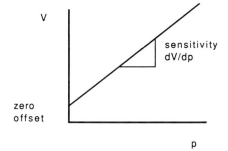

FIG. 1.2 Calibration curve showing zero offset and sensitivity, obtained by measuring p at two values and interpolating linearly.

another form, such as an electrical signal). The *input* is the quantity to be measured (for example, pressure, p), and the *output* is the signal (for example, voltage, V). A transducer is usually designed to be as linear as possible over the stated operating range, and to have very small *zero offset* and thus read "zero" when the input is zero. The transducer is calibrated by reading the mean output as the input is varied over the operating range. If this is impractical, but linearity can be assumed, measurements of the output can be made at two widely separated values on a standard. The linear calibration is then interpolated to any intermediate value. The slope dV/dp (change in output per unit change in input) is the *sensitivity*. The *nonlinearity* is the maximum input deviation from the straight line, divided by the full-scale input, and is usually expressed in a percentage.

Sensitivity and zero offset are subject to drift or change under environmental influences, such as change in temperature, and the measurement should be corrected for the difference in conditions from those prevailing during calibration. Many instruments are provided with a control to cancel the zero offset, so that zero output is achieved when the input is set to zero. An instrument may also be provided with a gain control to adjust the sensitivity of the system. Another source of error in some instruments is *hysteresis*. This is an effect in which the output depends on the previous history of the input variation; for example, whether the input was increasing or decreasing toward the point of interest. Hysteresis is characteristic of magnetic materials, backlash in gears, or any device in which energy is stored and not released completely. This effect can be measured by increasing and then decreasing the input. It is a good idea to vary the input in only one direction while making a series of measurements, and in the same direction during calibration.

The mean is best evaluated as the arithmetic average of a series of observations or measurements of the same quantity:

$$X = \frac{1}{n} \sum x_i \tag{1.1}$$

where X is the arithmetic average, x_i is the ith data point, n is the number of observations or measurements, and the summation is over i.

The deviation of the data point is $x_i - X$. The variance σ^2 is the average of the squares of the deviations, and the standard deviation is the square root of the variance:

$$\sigma = \sqrt{\frac{\sum (x_i - X)^2}{n - 1}}. \tag{1.2}$$

The sum is divided by $(n - 1)$ instead of n because one "degree of freedom" is used to determine the mean. The random error of the quantity measured is quoted as the standard deviation. The mean and standard deviation of a set of data points can be calculated by some pocket calculators, and the data need be entered only once.

For a large number of measurements, the probability of a certain deviation is given by the *normal distribution*, also termed the *Gaussian distribution*,

$$t = \frac{x - X}{\sigma'} \quad p(t) = \frac{1}{\sqrt{2n}} \exp\left[-\frac{t^2}{2}\right] \tag{1.3}$$

plotted in Fig. 1.3. By taking the area under the curve, it is found that 68.3 percent of the values should lie between 0 and plus or minus σ, 95.4 percent between 0 and plus or minus 2σ, and 99.7 percent between 0 and plus or minus 3σ.

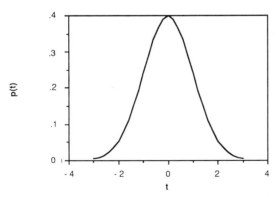

Average:

$$\bar{x} = \frac{1}{n} \sum_{i=1}^{n} x_i = X$$

Standard   deviation:

$$\sigma = \sqrt{\frac{\Sigma (x_i - \bar{x})^2}{n - 1}}$$

FIG. 1.3   Statistics. Normal or Gaussian distribution of probability against normalized deviation.

TABLE 1.2 Statistics

i	x_i	$x_i - X$	$(x_i - X)^2$
1	98	−3.4	11.56
2	110	8.6	93.96
3	99	−2.4	5.76
4	102	0.6	0.36
5	97	−4.4	19.36
6	95	−6.4	40.96
7	105	3.6	12.96
8	101	−0.4	0.16
9	114	12.6	158.76
10	93	−8.4	70.56
Σ	1014		414.4

$$\frac{\Sigma}{n} = \frac{1014}{10} \qquad\qquad \frac{\Sigma}{n-1} = \frac{414.4}{9}$$

$X = 101.4$ $\qquad\qquad\qquad \sigma^2 = 46.04$

Report as $X \pm \sigma = 101.4 \pm 6.8$ $\qquad \sigma = 6.79$

Results for 10 measurements of a quantity are listed in Table 1.2. Although they do not necessarily fit a Gaussian distribution exactly, it can be seen that the precision of these synthetic data is good.

When the mean Z of a third quantity is the sum or difference of two means, X and Y, the standard deviation is equal to the square root of the sum of the squares of the standard deviations of X and Y:

$$Z = X \pm Y, \sigma_z = \sqrt{\sigma_x^2 + \sigma_y^2}. \tag{1.4}$$

When the mean Z is given by the product or quotient of X and Y, the fractional standard deviation is equal to the square root of the sum of the fractional deviations squared of X and Y:

$$Z = XY \text{ or } X/Y, \frac{\sigma_z}{z} = \sqrt{\left(\frac{\sigma_x^2}{x}\right) + \left(\frac{\sigma_y^2}{y}\right)}. \tag{1.5}$$

Many measurements are subject to *background* and *noise*, which have to be subtracted. Background is the signal from an undesired input, and noise refers to the signal obtained when there is no input.

BIBLIOGRAPHY

Cobbold, R. S. C. 1974. *Transducers for biomedical measurements*, Wiley, New York: John Wiley & Sons.

Croxton, F. E. 1959. *Elementary statistics with applications in medicine and biological sciences. New York: Dover Publications.*

Dowdy, S., and S. Wearden. 1991. *Statistics for research.* 2d ed. John Wiley, New York: John Wiley & Sons.

Gylys, B. A., and M. E. Wedding. 1983. *Medical terminology.* Philadelphia: F.A. Davis.

Kapit, W., and L. M. Elson. 1977. *The anatomy coloring book.* New York: Harper & Row.

CHAPTER 2

HUMAN ANATOMY AND PHYSIOLOGY

2.0 CELLS, TISSUES, AND ORGANS

The human body is composed of specialized cells (organized into various tissues, which in turn constitute the different organs) and extracellular fibers and fluid. Organs are combined into systems to perform certain functions. This chapter is concerned with anatomy and aspects of physiology. There are many books on human anatomy and physiology, some of which are noted in the Bibliography at the end of this chapter. Only an overview is possible in this text; the references should be consulted for more detail.

A diagram of a generalized cell is shown in Fig. 2.1. Mammalian cells are eucaryotic: they contain a nucleus encapsulated in a porous nuclear membrane. The volume inside the nuclear membrane is filled with a viscous fluid (nucleoplasm), the genetic material (DNA plus protein, organized into chromosomes or dispersed as chromatin), and one or more nucleoli (singular, *nucleolus*), which produce RNA. The entire cell is contained within the cell (plasma) membrane, which has many functions in addition to separating the cell from the extracellular environment. In addition to the cytoplasm filling the cell, there are vacuoles and pinocytic or phagocytic vesicles involved in intake, elimination, or storage of liquids and solids. There are many organelles embedded in the cytoplasm. The endoplasmic reticulum (ER) consists of layers of flattened vesicles involved in transport of proteins and other chemicals. Granular or rough ER is covered with small bodies called *ribosomes*, where RNA directs the assembly of amino acids into various proteins, including enzymes. The Golgi complex is associated with secretion. Lysosomes are containers for enzymes that destroy cell debris or foreign manner in the vacuoles. Mitochondria are membrane-lined organelles with enzymes, in-

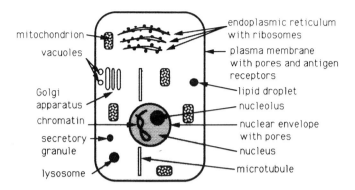

FIG. 2.1 Schematic diagram of generalized animal cell.

volved in cell "respiration" (utilization of oxygen and production of carbon dioxide and the energy-storing chemical ATP [adenosine triphosphate]). Microtubules and fibrils provide a type of skeleton for the cell and, with the centrioles, are involved in cell movement and in mitosis and cell division. The surfaces of some cells are equipped with flagella (for motion), cilia (for movement of material past the cell), or microvilli (for increased absorption surface).

Body cells are specialized to perform certain functions. For example, although all cells secrete various substances, glandular cells are specialized for secretion; most cells can change shape, but muscle cells are specialized for contraction; and so forth. The mature erythrocyte (red blood cell [RBC]) is unusual in that it lacks a nucleus. It is specialized to transport oxygen in combination with hemoglobin and is basically a membrane filled with fluid containing hemoglobin.

Cells are organized into four types of tissues: epithelial, connective, muscle, and nervous. Examples of tissues and specialized cells are shown in Fig. 2.2. The types of epithelial tissues are identified by the morphology of the cells, for example, flattened and scalelike (squamous), cuboidal, columnar; as simple (single-layer) or stratified (multilayer); by the presence or absence of cilia on the free surface of the tissue; and by function (e.g., secretion of hormones by exocrine or endocrine glands). Simple squamous epithelium lines all blood and lymphatic vessels, alveoli (air sacs) of the lungs, and some kidney tubules. It is adapted for diffusion and filtration. Cuboidal and columnar cells line glands and the digestive tract and are involved in secretion and absorption. Pseudostratified columnar epithelium lines the respiratory tract. Its glands secrete mucus and its cilia move mucus and particles out of the lungs. Stratified squamous epithelium lines the skin, oral cavity, and much of the pharynx, esophagus, vagina, and anal canal; it is primarily protective. Stratified columnar epithelium lines part of the reproductive tract. The urinary bladder, ureter, and kidneys contain transitional epithelium that can expand or contract according to the volume of urine. Exocrine (ducted) glands are pockets lined

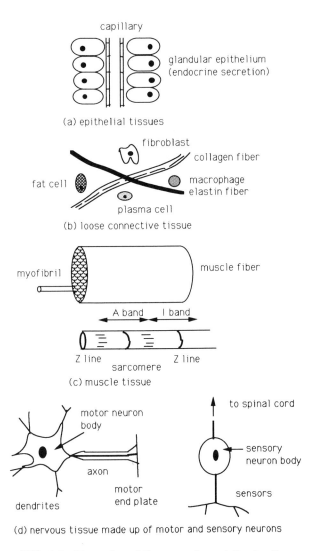

FIG. 2.2   Examples of tissues and specialized cells.

with epithelial cells that secrete mucus, serous fluid (similar to blood plasma), sebaceous (oily) fluid, sweat (slightly saline water), milk, and so on. Endocrine (ductless) glands secrete hormones into the blood.

Connective tissues include blood, connective tissues proper (fibrous, elastic, adipose) and the supporting tissues, cartilage, and bone. Blood and blood cells are discussed in greater detail in Section 2.3, and cartilage and bone in Section 2.2. Fibrous tissue may be loose or dense. Loose or areolar tissue consists of a viscous, amorphous, carbohydrate-protein matrix, a loose and irregular mesh of collagen and elastin fibers, plus various kinds of cells.

Fibroblasts secrete collagen (a protein of high tensile strength) and elastin (an elastic protein). Fat cells store fat. Macrophages, which engulf bacteria and other foreign matter, are able to move through the matrix. Plasma cells, lymphocytes, and other white blood cells (WBCs [leukocytes]) are also motile and are part of the immune system. Loose connective tissue is found under the skin; it supports the epithelia of viscera and cavities and generally fills spaces throughout the body. Adipose tissue consists predominantly of fat cells, along with some fibers and capillaries; it is located around some viscera, under the skin, and elsewhere. Adipose tissue serves as a store of fat for energy, insulation, and protective padding. Dense regular (aligned fiber) tissue consists of collagen fibers and fibroblasts; this type of tissue constitutes tendons and ligaments. Dense irregular fibrous tissue includes an irregular mat of collagen, elastin fibers, and fibroblasts, encapsulates certain organs, cartilage, and bone, and supports the epithelial layer of the skin (dermis). Elastic tissue consists mainly of elastic fibers and a few fibroblasts; it is found in arterial walls, some veins, alveoli of the lungs, and elsewhere. Reticular fibers are small collagen fibers in a loose array; they support liver cells, lymphatic tissue cells, and cells in the bone marrow.

The muscle cells are long and spindle shaped and have a centrally located nucleus. Visceral muscle is smooth (with no transverse bands or striations). Smooth muscle is found in the walls of cavities in viscera such as the digestive tract, urinary tract, respiratory tract, reproductive system ducts, and blood vessels. It moves or controls the flow of material along the length of the cavity by slow, rhythmic contractions. Most smooth muscle contracts in response to hormonal as well as nervous stimulation, but is not under voluntary control. Cardiac muscle cells have striations, junctions between cells (intercalated discs), a centrally located nucleus, and split or bifurcated ends. Contraction is initiated by special electrical-impulse–conducting muscle cells, but the heart rate is regulated by the autonomic nervous system (not under voluntary control). Cardiac muscle makes up the wall of the heart (myocardium). Skeletal muscle is striated, long, and cylindrical (10 to 100 μm in diameter, up to 4 cm long) and the cells ("fibers") contain several nuclei. Skeletal muscle, which is under voluntary control, moves the bones.

Each muscle cell contains many myofibrils, which in turn are made up of myofilaments of actin and myosin. The actin filaments are anchored to a structure called the Z line at one end of the functional unit called a *sarcomere*. During contraction, the thin actin filaments slide between the thicker, fixed myosin filaments, making and breaking cross-bridges. The energy is provided by the breakdown of ATP into ADP and phosphate. Continuous contraction is prevented by two regulator proteins, troponin and tropomyosin. However, the blocking is stopped by calcium ion, controlled by the nervous system. The combined effect of the sliding in the many sarcomeres results in the muscle's contracting about one-third of its resting length. The maximum contraction force is exerted at the resting length. More information on muscle is given in Chapter 4.

The basic unit of the nervous system is the nerve cell, or neuron. There is a cell body with its nucleus and its processes (axon and dendrites). A neuron with one process (e.g., sensory cells) is called unipolar. A neuron with two processes (axon and dendrite) is bipolar, and one with many processes is multipolar. An axon conducts impulses away from the cell body, whereas dendrites receive and conduct impulses toward the cell body. The insulating myelin (phospholipid) sheath is formed by the coiling of a special cell, the Schwann cell, around the cell process. There are gaps, called nodes of Ranvier, about 1 mm apart, between the Schwann cells. The outside of the Schwann cell is the neurilemma. Where myelin is absent, as in some parts of the central nervous system (CNS), the neurilemma is provided by supporting cells called *glia*. The cell body contains the nucleus and Nissl granules, which are involved in protein synthesis.

The mechanism of the generation of the action potential in a neuron is illustrated in Fig. 2.3. Active chemical processes cause an accumulation of

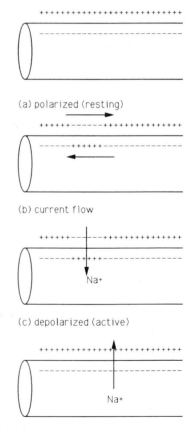

(a) polarized (resting)

(b) current flow

(c) depolarized (active)

(d) repolarization

FIG. 2.3 Mechanism of generation of the nerve action potential.

Na^+ ions on the outside of the cell membrane, and an accumulation of K^+ ions on the inside. In the resting cell, the membrane is more impermeable to Na^+ and more permeable to K^+, leading to a slow leakage of K^+ out of the cell, an accumulation of excess positive charge (both ions) outside, and a difference in potential across the cell membrane (resting potential) on the order of -70 mV. When a neuron is stimulated, the cell membrane at that point becomes about 500 times more permeable to Na^+ ions, which flow into the cell, creating a measurable electrical charge, the action potential. Potassium ions move more slowly out of the cell. The potential of the cell becomes reversed (to about $+40$ mV), the inside becoming positive to the outside, and the cell is depolarized. A depolarized area of cell membrane thus lies adjacent to a polarized area, and a current flows between the two areas. Newly depolarized areas are formed, and the nerve impulse propagates down the axon of the neuron at about 45 cm/sec. Depolarization is followed by repolarization about 3 ms after the current flow, because of the action of the sodium-potassium pump. In myelinated neurons, the current flow takes place at the nodes between the myelin sheaths, so that depolarization occurs in a series of jumps, and nerve impulse propagation is hundreds of times faster than in unmyelinated neurons. Once a neuron is stimulated to generate an action potential, it cannot generate another action potential for some 10 to 15 ms (refractory period) unless the stimulus is much greater.

Neurons communicate with each other or with a muscle cell through a synapse. Action potentials may be either excitatory or inhibitory at a synapse. Signals (nerve impulses) are transmitted across the synaptic cleft by chemicals called *neurotransmitters*. Neurotransmitters include acetylcholine; monamines such as dopamine, norepinephrine, and epinephrine; certain amino acids and related chemicals such as GABA (gamma-aminobutyric acid, an inhibitory neurotransmitter); and various peptides.

2.1 INTEGUMENTARY SYSTEM

The integument is the skin and related structures (hair, nails, glands). Skin envelops and protects the entire body, grading into mucous membrane at body openings. The integument is important for controlling loss of fluids and contributes to temperature regulation (by evaporation of sweat, erection of hair, and shivering). It is the largest organ of the body, constituting about 7 percent of body weight, and has a surface area of some 1.8 m² in the adult. Average thickness is 1 to 2 mm, but the thickness varies from 6 mm on the palms, soles, and back to 0.5 mm on the eyelid. The skin comprises an epithelial layer, the epidermis, and a connective tissue layer, the dermis. The dermis in turn is supported by the superficial fascia.

The epidermis varies in thickness from 0.07 to 0.12 mm over most of the body, to 0.8 mm on the palms and 1.4 mm on the soles. The epidermis consists of the stratum corneum (a keratinous layer of dead squamous cells), the stratum lucidum and stratum granulosum (evident only in thick skin), the stratum spinosum, and the stratum basale, from which all the outer cells arise. Cells in the latter two layers are actively dividing and make up for the loss of cells at the skin surface. The cells of the stratum spinosum, or the Malpighi layer, contain varying amounts of melanin particles, the brown pigment produced by melanocytes. Melanin serves to protect against ultraviolet light (sunlight) and gives the characteristic color of the skin. Merkel's discs, nerve endings specialized for touch, also extend into the epidermis.

The dermis consists of an outer, soft papillary layer and an inner reticular layer of collagenous fibers. The papillae are projections into the epidermis, which, when regularly arranged, provide friction ridges—hence fingerprints. Many papillae contain capillaries to nourish the epidermal layers, and some contain nerves with special endings for the sensation of touch (Meissner's corpuscles). The reticular layer contains fibers, nerves (with specialized endings for sensing pain, touch, heat, and cold), arteries and veins, lymphatic vessels, and sweat glands. Hair grows from a matrix in the bulb of the hair follicle. Associated with the follicle is a blood supply (in the dermal papilla), a sebaceous gland, and an arrector pili muscle that erects hair for better insulation.

The dermis grades into the superficial fascia, or hypodermis, a layer of loose connective tissue including adipose tissue and the pacinian capsules, sensors of pressure and vibration. Some voluntary muscles may also be present. Blood vessels, lymphatics, and nerves traverse the subcutaneous layer on the way to the dermis and epidermis. The superficial fascia is usually thicker than the dermis.

2.2   SKELETAL-MUSCULAR SYSTEMS

The skeletal system is made of cartilage and bone, with joints allowing movement. In addition to movement, bone provides support, protection of soft tissues, a place for blood cell production, and a storehouse for calcium. The 206 bones in the human skeleton are classified as long (such as the femur and other bones of the limbs), short (ankle and wrist bones), flat (skull, ribs, and sternum), and irregular (vertebral column, pelvis, clavicle, etc.), and amount to 18 percent of body mass.

During development, most bone starts as hyaline cartilage, a connective tissue consisting of a gelatinous organic matrix interspersed with collagenous fibers and the matrix-secreting chondrocytes. Cartilage lacks blood vessels, except in the surrounding fibrous sheath. In the adult, hyaline cartilage is found in the nose, larynx, part of the rib cage, and caps at the ends of bones. Elastic cartilage, which is hyaline cartilage with elastic fibers, is found in the epiglottis and the external ear. Fibrocartilage includes collagen fibers and is located in the discs between vertebrae and other bones, and in joint capsules and ligaments that bind joints together. Cartilage is tough and strong, but flexible.

Bone is a well-engineered structural material, combining strength, rigidity, and low weight. The mechanical properties of bone are listed in Table 2.1. A typical bone has two regions, one in which the bone matter is dense or compact and another in which it is spongy or cancellous and, therefore, of reduced weight. Compact bone is located on the outside, where it is most efficiently used to withstand various forces, especially bending. There is a thin layer of compact bone on the end (epiphysis) and a thicker layer in the shaft (diaphysis). The cancellous portion is made up of threads or trabeculae, which are arranged according to lines of tension and compression. The hollow space inside many bones is filled with red marrow (part of the hemopoietic or blood-cell–forming system) or fatty, yellow marrow. Bone matter itself is a composite, with some 60 percent by volume (and 40 percent by weight) composed of the organic, rubbery collagen and the rest made up of micro-crystals of calcium hydroxyapatite $(Ca_{10}(PO_4)_6(OH)_2)$. Normal compact bone has a density of 1.9 g/cm^3, of which 22 weight percent is calcium, an efficient absorber of x-rays and low-energy gamma rays because of its relatively large atomic number (20). Calcium may be gained or lost, depending on diet and the demands of the body for calcium ion.

Bone is a living organ, allowing for growth and for remodeling by osteoclasts (cells that break down bone) and osteoblasts (cells that build bone). Bone is provided with a blood supply by blood vessels and nerves located in the haversian canals leading to small fluid cavities (lacunae) containing osteocytes. The entire bone, except for the cartilage in joints, is covered by the periosteum, a fibrous and vascular membrane with numerous cells. In the human body up to age 20 to 25, the epiphysis is separated from the diaphysis by a cartilage plate. Growth proceeds from both the epiphysis and the diaphysis until all cartilage is replaced by bone and growth ceases.

In a joint, the ends of the bone are covered by cartilage. A synovial fluid is secreted by and contained within a synovial membrane. Synovial fluid contains water, hyaluronic acid, and high molecular weight mucopolysaccharides, has the consistency of egg white, and acts as a lubricant. The coefficient of friction is less than 0.01, better than that of a skate blade on ice. Joints are classified according to the degree of freedom or motion permitted, as well as the shape and fit of the bones. A hinge joint, such as the elbow, allows motion about one axis only, at right angles to the bones. Pivot joints, such as those in the neck vertebrae, allow movement around an axis through

TABLE 2.1   Mechanical Properties of Compact Bone

Tensile strength	120 N/mm^2
Compressive strength	170 N/mm^2
Young's modulus	1.8×10^4 N/mm^2

the bones. Condyloid joints, as in the wrist, are biaxial and permit flexion-extension and rotation. Saddle joints, as in the thumb, are also biaxial. Ball-and-socket joints are universal joints, allowing motion in many directions around a fixed center. The shoulder and hip are ball-and-socket joints. An artificial ball-and-socket (hip) joint is discussed in Chapter 4. Nerves ending in the joint capsule are part of the proprioception system, which signals the position and orientation of the bones.

Muscle makes up some 40 percent of body mass. Some muscles are used primarily for maintaining posture, whereas others are involved in movement. A muscle may be partially contracted but not moving, and hence isometric (at a constant length). The metabolic (ATP) energy derived from digestion of food is converted into heat. Because muscle is elastic but can exert a force only while contracting, movement is effected by contracting one muscle (the agonist) and relaxing the opposing muscle (antagonist). The reverse movement is achieved by relaxing the first muscle and contracting the opposing one. In flexing the arm, the biceps is the agonist and the triceps is the antagonist, whereas in extending the arm the roles are reversed. If a muscle is contracting and moving against weight or resistance, it is said to have isotonic action, and metabolic energy is converted into mechanical work at about 40 percent efficiency, the rest manifested as heat. The maximum pulling force per unit of cross-sectional area is about 3.1×10^7 N/m^2, exerted when the muscle is at its resting length. Muscle is well supplied with blood to deliver nutrients and oxygen and to remove waste products and heat. Metabolic energy is provided by ATP, which is generated in the mitochondria; thus, muscle cells contain many mitochondria. Glycogen granules also provide a store of chemical energy. Motor nerves stimulate the muscle cells, either directly or through conduction by other muscle cells. Sensory nerves detect velocity and extension of the muscles, and the coordination of movement is achieved in the cerebellum of the brain. Muscles are enveloped in fibrous connective tissue, the fascia. Additional information about muscles may be found in Chapter 4.

2.3 CIRCULATORY SYSTEM

The circulatory system includes the cardiovascular system and the lymphatic system. The cardiovascular system consists of the heart (a pump), the arteries and smaller arterioles that carry blood away from the heart, the capillaries, and the small venules and larger veins that carry blood back to the heart. These form complete circuits to carry blood throughout the body, which are diagrammed in Fig. 2.4. In the main systemic circulation, oxygenated blood leaves the left ventricle of the heart under pressure and passes through the aorta and other arteries to the capillaries in the upper and lower parts of the body. A branch goes to the digestive tract and the liver (portal circulation). The deoxygenated blood returns through the veins at low pressure to the

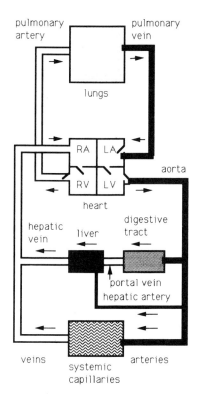

FIG. 2.4 Schematic of circulatory system. Oxygenated blood in vessels is shown black, nonoxygenated blood as white.

right atrium of the heart. Pulmonary circulation proceeds from the right ventricle to the lungs, where the blood takes up oxygen (and releases carbon dioxide) and then returns to the left atrium and left ventricle of the heart. Blood transports not only oxygen, but also nutrients, water, and hormones to the cells, cellular waste products (including carbon dioxide) to the lungs, and urea to the kidneys. Blood also aids in regulation of body temperature and is involved in the immune function by transporting WBCs and antibodies.

Some properties of blood in the average healthy adult are listed in Table 2.2. Blood is a fluid with suspended cells: the erthrocytes (RBCs) that transport oxygen, the leucocytes (WBCs) involved in immunity, and thrombocytes or platelets that participate in blood clotting. The noncellular component of blood, called *plasma*, is composed of 91 percent water, 7 percent plasma proteins (albumin, globulin, prothrombin, and fibrinogen), 0.9 percent electrolytes (sodium, potassium, calcium, and magnesium chlorides, bicarbonates, and sulfates or phosphates), and many other substances, including nutrients (glucose, amino acids, fatty acids, and vitamins), waste (including carbon dioxide, mostly as bicarbonate, urea, and uric acid), hormones, and antibodies. The hematocrit, or packed cell volume, is the percentage of erythrocytes by volume and can be measured by centrifuging heparinized blood (to prevent clotting) or waiting for the cells to settle in a vertical tube. The

TABLE 2.2 Properties of Normal Blood

Volume	5–6 liters (8% of body weight)
Hematocrit	40–47% of total volume
Red cell count	5×10^6 per mm^3
White cell count	8×10^3 per mm^3 total
	5200 neutrophils
	320 eosinophils
	80 basophils
	2000 lymphocytes
	400 monocytes
Platelet count	2.5×10^5 per mm^3
Hemoglobin	0.145 g per ml
pH	7.4
Specific gravity	1.055

WBCs and platelets form a thin layer, the "buffy coat" on top of the RBCs, about 1 percent of whole blood volume.

RBCs, formed from stem cells in the bone marrow, have a lifetime of 120 days and must be replaced continuously. An unconstrained, normal erythrocyte is a biconcave disc 7.2 mm in diameter and 2.2 mm thick at the rim. It contains hemoglobin, a compound of 4 heme groups (containing one atom each of ferrous iron and able to loosely bind oxygen) and the protein globin, with a molecular weight of 67,000. One gram of hemoglobin is able to combine with 1.34 ml of oxygen (at normal pressure and temperature). When combined with oxygen (that is, oxygenated), the compound is called *oxyhemoglobin* and the blood is bright red. When deoxygenated (deoxyhemoglobin), blood is dark blue. In abnormal conditions, when the lungs do not reoxygenate the blood fully, even arterial blood is blue and the subject becomes visibly blue, or cyanotic. Normally, blood leaves the lungs with 95 to 100 percent oxyhemoglobin. It returns to the lungs with 70 percent oxyhemoglobin. Thus, on average, only 25 to 30 percent of the available oxygen is used. In the basal (completely resting) state, the body requires about 250 ml of oxygen per minute. The blood flow is 5 to 6 l per minute, hence the average organ consumes 40 ml of oxygen per liter of blood. The heart muscle, however, requires some 110 ml of oxygen per liter, and the brain also has higher-than-average oxygen demand. The kidneys receive a much greater flow than required for their metabolism, because they "filter" the blood, and oxygen demand per liter is much lower than average. Skeletal muscle also uses less than average amounts of oxygen, except when exercising. Skin is overperfused because the blood also serves to reject heat.

WBCs are of various types: granulocytes (neutrophils, eosinophils, and basophils, which stain differently), lymphocytes, and monocytes. Granulocytes originate from stem cells in the bone marrow and live only a few days. Neutrophils are phagocytic, eosinophils proliferate in allergic reactions, and basophils are circulating mast cells that produce heparin and histamine. Lymphocytes originate in myeloid (bone marrow) and lymphoid tissues and live a few days to 200 days. Monocytes are phagocytic and are formed in the bone marrow.

Platelets are parts of particular cells. They aggregate and break down at a site of injury or foreign surface, releasing the vasoconstrictor serotonin. Tissue damage or breakdown of platelets releases thromboplastin (thrombokinase), an enzyme that facilitates, in the presence of calcium ion, the conversion of the plasma protein prothrombin into thrombin. Thrombin is a protein-splitting enzyme that breaks down the plasma protein fibrogen into smaller units, which then polymerize into the insoluble protein fibrin. Fibrin forms sticky threads that trap blood cells and form a clot. The initially soft clot contracts in about 10 minutes and exudes serum (i.e., plasma without the cells, fibrinogen, and other factors involved in clotting). The process is actually more complicated than described, and several other substances (factors) are involved, whereby a deficiency can result in impaired clotting.

A thrombus is a clot occurring in the cardiovascular system, which produces a condition called *thrombosis*. A thrombus in the arteries supplying the heart muscle (coronary thrombosis) blocks the artery and may be fatal. A thrombus may form when a change, such as roughening or injury, occurs in the smooth endothelial lining of a blood vessel or in the heart. A thrombus that becomes detached is called an *embolus*. An embolus that becomes lodged in the lung may be especially serious. Manufactured materials such as plastics are not as smooth as the body's own endothelium. Therefore, part of the challenge in using engineering devices such as an artificial heart, a heart-lung bypass machine, or any extracorporeal blood circuit is to avoid formation of a thrombus or embolus. The clotting tendency can be reduced by the administration of anticoagulant drugs such as heparin. Blood collected for later transfusion is taken from a vein with minimum tissue damage, transferred into a silicone-lined or other smooth tube or vessel and mixed in the vessel with acid sodium citrate and dextrose. The citrate removes calcium ions by forming calcium citrate, so that clotting will not occur, and the dextrose serves as food for the red cells. The blood is stored at 4°C and lasts about 3 weeks before too many red cells are hemolysed.

The heart is a muscular organ about the size of a clenched fist, or 12 cm long, 9 cm wide, tapering to an apex, and 6 cm thick. It is located between the lungs (in the mediastinum) in the anterior inferior part of the thoracic (chest) cavity, between the second and fifth intercostal spaces, with two-thirds of the mass on the left side. It is contained in a sac of parietal pericardium attached to the inside of the sternal wall and to the diaphragm. As indicated in Fig. 2.5, the heart is divided into four chambers: right atrium, right ventricle, left atrium, and left ventricle. The right side of the heart pumps blood to the lungs, and the left side pumps blood to the rest of the body. A system of valves prevents backflow. The most important valves in the adult are the atrioventricular valves (the tricuspid valve between the right atrium and ven-

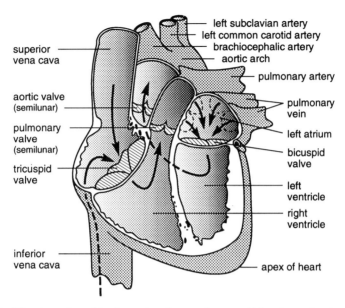

superior
vena cava

aortic valve
(semilunar)

pulmonary
valve
(semilunar)

tricuspid
valve

inferior
vena cava

left subclavian artery
left common carotid artery
brachiocephalic artery
aortic arch

pulmonary artery

pulmonary
vein

left atrium

bicuspid
valve

left
ventricle

right
ventricle

apex of heart

FIG. 2.5 Heart, sectioned to show chambers, valves, and blood vessels. *Arrows* show direction of blood flow.

tricle and the bicuspid valve between the left atrium and ventricle) and the semilunar valves (in the aorta and pulmonary artery).

The heart walls consist of an inner endocardium, middle myocardium, and outer epicardium. The endocardium has an endothelium layer lining the chambers and valves and continuous with the blood vessels, and a fibrous layer for support. The endocardium supports blood vessels and electrical-impulse–conducting tissue. The myocardium is the variable thickness layer of cardiac muscle, up to 2.5 cm thick at the left ventricle, where most of the work in pumping blood is performed. The arrangement of the muscle fibers produces a wringing motion that empties the ventricles. The inner myocardium is irregular in shape, with papillae and trabeculae. The myocardium is permeated by capillaries and lymphatics and a rich supply of oxygenated blood. The epicardium is a thin, transparent layer of fibrous tissue with an outer covering of mesoepithelium. It has blood vessels, lymphatics, and fat. The parietal pericardium, consisting of an inner serous coat and outer fibrous coat, completely encloses the heart and the bases of the blood vessels. The space between the pericardium and the epicardium is lubricated by a watery fluid.

The heartbeat is automatic, independent of the nervous system. It is controlled by the sinoatrial (S-A) node of specialized muscle tissue, located at the entrance to the right atrium. Electrical impulses travel through special cardiac muscle cells in the myocardium to the atrial walls, causing them to contract simultaneously. Another mass of tissue, the atrioventricular (A-V) node in the right atrium, receives the atrial impulse, delays it, and transmits an impulse through the atrioventricular bundle (bundle of His) into the septum between the ventricles, where it divides into right and left branches. The branches divide into Purkinje fibers, which terminate in contractile muscle cells. The electrical impulse stimulates the ventricular contraction, starting at the apex and driving the blood out of the ventricle. If this conducting system should fail (heart block), the atria will beat faster than the ventricles, and all independently. When properly conducting and coordinated, the heart will pump blood at about 50 percent mechanical efficiency, 72 beats per minute (resting), for a lifetime.

The pumping cycle begins with the heart relaxed, the semilunar valves closed, the atrioventricular valves open, and the atria filling with blood. At the next stage (diastole), the atria are contracting, ventricles are relaxed and filling, semilunar valves remain closed, and atrioventricular valves remain open. In the following stage (systole), the atria are relaxed while the ventricles contract, the semilunar valves are open and the atrioventricular valves closed, and blood is pumped into the pulmonary artery and aorta. The cycle then begins again. The ventricular stroke volume is about 75 ml, hence at 70 to 80 beats per minute the cardiac output is 5 to 6 liters per minute at a left ventricle pressure of 120 torr. More information on the heart may be found in Chapter 3 and 4.

Arteries range in diameter from about 25 mm (aorta) to about 0.5 mm. The thin inner layer (tunica intima) consists of smooth endothelium with a basement membrane and some connective tissue. The thick intermediate layer (tunica media) is composed of smooth muscle and elastic connective tissue, usually arranged circumferentially. The thinner outer layer (tunica externa or adventitia) contains fibrous connective tissue and a few muscle fibers, arranged longitudinally. Artery walls are elastic, smoothing out the blood flow and lowering peak blood pressure by stretching. In arteriosclerosis (hardening of the arteries) elasticity is lost and the blood pressure is raised. Arterioles are defined as arteries of less than 0.5 mm in diameter. They are lined with endothelial cells, and their walls are more muscular than elastic. Muscular arterioles help control blood flow to the capillaries; they also contract spastically if injured, which protects against major hemorrhaging. If the main artery or arteriole serving a certain volume is occluded, it can sometimes be replaced by new arterioles that establish a collateral circulation. If circulation is lost entirely, the tissue in the region dies (an infarct).

A capillary is about 1 mm long and 8 to 10 μm in diameter, about the size of an RBC. It consist of a single layer of endothelial cells, which may be backed by a basement membrane and loose connective tissue containing tissue fluid. The capillaries form a fine network, such that every cell is within about 100 μm of a capillary. Not all of the capillaries are patent (open) at once; instead, some close and then open again. The flow is controlled by muscle sphincters at the junction of the capillary and the arteriole or by muscle fibers along the capillary. Some "thoroughfare" channels connect the arteriole and the venule more or less directly, whereas true capillaries tend to branch and join or interconnect (anatomose). The capillary network, or bed, forms the microvasculature, where materials are exchanged between blood and the cells.

Venules are similar to large capillaries, but their walls have some fibrous tissue and a few muscle fibers. Veins have walls similar to those of arteries, but the layers are less well defined and the tunica media may be absent. Veins are on the low-pressure side of the capillary bed and thus do not have to be as strong as arteries. Because of the low pressure and slow flow, veins may be larger in diameter or there may be more veins than arteries. Backflow prevention valves are located in veins, such as those in the legs, which have to carry blood against gravity back to the heart. The contraction of surrounding skeletal muscles helps to force blood upward. There are no valves in the veins of the pulmonary and portal circulation, or in the arteries.

The lymphatic system includes the lymphatic capillaries and lymphatic vessels, lymph nodes, spleen, thymus,and tonsils. This is not a closed circulatory system, but one that collects interstitial tissue fluid and returns it to the blood. Lymph capillaries in the intestinal villi absorb fats from the digestive system. Lymph nodes are filters; they also process lymphocytes, which are part of the immune system. The other organs in the lymphatic system are also part of the immune system.

2.4 RESPIRATORY SYSTEM

The respiratory system consists of the lungs and the airways transporting air to and from them: the nasal cavity, the pharynx, the larynx, the trachea, and the bronchi. The major function of the respiratory system is to exchange oxygen and carbon dioxide with the blood. The system also includes the olfactory organ (for the sense of smell) and the vocal folds (vocal cords) in the larynx. Small amounts of heat and moisture are lost from the body through the expired air.

On inspiration, air is drawn into the nasal cavity, which is divided into left and right sides and has "shelves," or conchae. The cavity and other conducting passages are lined with pseudostratified columnar ciliated epithelium that has many goblet cells that secrete mucus. The cilia work to sweep dust and other particles out of the respiratory tract. The olfactory cells are located at the top of the nasal cavity. Various passages communicate with the sinuses in the skull, and the Eustachian tube equalizes pressure in the inner ear. Air is warmed and saturated with moisture during its passage through the airways. The respiratory tract is well supplied with lymphatic tissue to defend against inhaled bacteria and other matter.

The inhaled air passes through the pharynx, which is shared with the digestive system. During swallowing, the larynx is sealed off by a flap of cartilage, the epiglottis. When the epiglottis is open, air flows into the larynx, a tube reinforced by cartilage rings. The vocal folds (or cords) are ligaments lined with mucosa (epithelium), stretching between two movable cartilages, under muscular control, to abduct or adduct the folds (opening or closing the air passage between them) and thus initiate sounds on expiration.

Beyond the larynx, the air flows through the trachea, thence to the right and left main bronchi, and further subdividing many times into progressively smaller diameter bronchi (serving the lobes and segments of the lungs), then to the bronchioles, alveoli ducts, and, finally, the actual respiratory units (the respiratory duct, the alveolar duct, and the tiny air sacs, the alveoli). The bronchial tree and respiratory unit are shown in Fig. 2.6. The trachea is a tube, about 2.5 cm in diameter and 11 cm long, of fibrous tissue reinforced by C-shaped cartilage rings, so that it cannot collapse, and lined with the respiratory epithelium. It lies anteriorly to the esophagus. The bronchi are of similar construction. Walls are lined with mucosa (pseudostratified columnar ciliated epithelium with goblet cells, with a basement membrane on

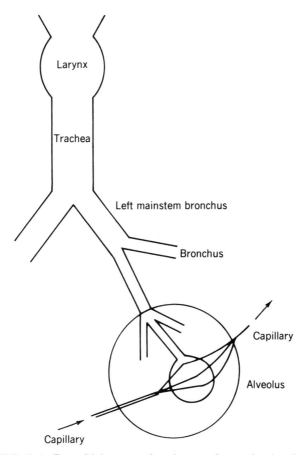

FIG. 2.6 Bronchial tract and exchange of gases in alveolus.

fibrous tissue containing many lymphocytes, small blood and lymph vessels, and nerves). The submucosa is made of fibrous connective tissue with larger blood vessels and glands. Bronchioles are distinguished by their small diameter (1 mm or less), the absence of cartilage, and smooth muscle and elastic tissue in their walls.

The actual exchange of oxygen and carbon dioxide occurs between the gases dissolved in water and diffusing through the single-cell layer of the alveolar wall and the blood in capillaries enveloping the alveolus (respiratory unit). There are some 300 million alveoli in the human lung, with a gas exchange surface of 70 to 80 m². Their collapse is prevented by a coating of phospholipid surfactant that reduces surface tension. The pulmonary veins and arteries enter the lung at the hilus and subdivide to the alveolar capillaries. About three-fifths of the lung volume is blood and blood vessels. Oxygen exchange occurs because of differences in the partial pressures on each side of the alveolar-capillary wall. These pressures are given in Table 2.3. The air is saturated with water vapor at body temperature (37°C). There is less oxygen and more carbon dioxide in alveolar than in atmospheric air, because oxygen is transferred *to* blood and carbon dioxide *from* blood. If the alveoli are ventilated more strongly in breathing, carbon dioxide is "blown off" and exits the body, thus reducing the partial pressure of carbon dioxide in the alveoli as compared with that of the deoxygenated blood in the capillary. Because the total pressure has to remain the same, and the nitrogen and saturated water vapor pressures do not change much, the oxygen pressure is increased over that in the blood, and more oxygen combines with hemoglobin. The process is controlled with a setpoint for carbon dioxide pressure and the pH of the blood, sensed by cells in the brainstem.

Figure 2.7a plots the oxygen dissociation curve and partial pressure of oxygen throughout the cardiovascular system. At oxygen partial pressures above 100 mm Hg the hemoglobin is fully saturated. For a normal hemoglobin concentration of 14.5 g/100 ml of blood, and normal carbon dioxide concentration, the oxygen capacity is 20 ml oxygen/100 ml of blood. After passing through the tissues, the oxygen partial pressure is reduced to 40 mm Hg. In the lung, the partial pressure is raised again to 100 mm Hg.

Figure 2.7b plots the carbon dioxide dissociation curve and the partial pressure throughout the cardiovascular system. The partial pressure is 46 mm Hg (torr) in the tissues and blood until the blood passes through the lungs.

TABLE 2.3   Partial Pressures of Air Components, torr

	Atmosphere	Alveoli
Nitrogen	600	563
Water vapor	varies	47
Oxygen	159	110
Carbon dioxide	1	40

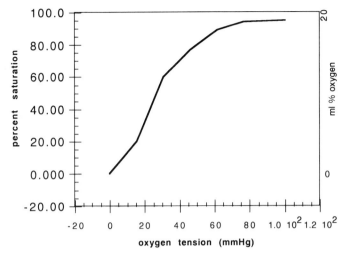

FIG. 2.7a Oxygen dissociation curve. Arterial point is 100 mm Hg with 95 percent saturation, and venous point is 40 mm Hg at 70 percent saturation. 1 mm Hg = 1 torr.

There the partial pressure is lowered to 40 mm Hg (torr). Most CO_2 is carried as bicarbonate, and there is no saturation. The content is 48 to 52 ml CO_2 per 100 ml of blood.

The lungs are essentially passive in breathing. They are enclosed in pleura, membranes with serous fluid between them, for low friction. A negative pressure (relative to atmospheric) is produced in the lung when the chest cavity expands. Expansion, hence inspiration, occurs when the vagus nerve

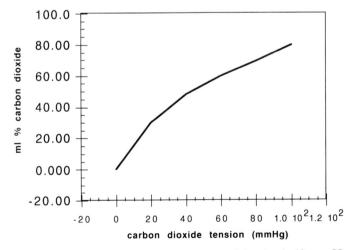

FIG. 2.7b Carbon dioxide dissociation curve. Arterial point is 40 mm Hg at 48 ml percent (ml gas per 100 ml blood); venous point is 46 mm Hg at 52 ml percent. 1 mm Hg = 1 torr.

stimulates the contraction of the diaphragm (which flattens it) and the rib cage is raised by the intercostal muscles. Expiration occurs through the natural elasticity of the lungs and the relaxation of the diaphragm and rib muscles. Not all of the air is expelled. The tidal volume that is breathed in and out is 500 ml, of which 150 ml is dead space in the airways. Resting, the respiration rate is 14 breaths per minute, corresponding to about 5 liters per minute, in the adult. The total lung capacity is the volume with the maximum full breath taken in (3.9 to 9.4 liters in the male, 2.5 to 6.9 liters in the female). The functional residual capacity is the volume with the respiratory muscles fully relaxed, which is about 40 percent of the lung capacity. If an effort is made to forcibly expel air, one reaches the residual capacity, about 20 percent of the total lung capacity. More information may be found in Chapters 3 and 4.

2.5   DIGESTIVE SYSTEM

The digestive system consists of the alimentary canal (oral cavity with teeth and tongue, pharynx, esophagus, stomach, small intestine, large intestine, and rectum) and glands that produce digestive juices, including enzymes (salivary glands, stomach lining, pancreas, liver, gall bladder, and intestinal secretions). An overall view of the system is shown in Fig. 2.8. The principal function of the digestive system is to break down food into simple nutrients (e.g., glucose, fatty acids, amino acids) that can be used by cells and to absorb the nutrients (including vitamins and minerals) into the bloodstream. Un-

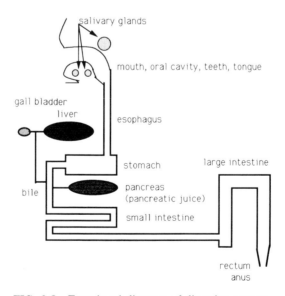

FIG. 2.8   Functional diagram of digestive system.

usable substances, along with shed cells, bacteria, and other waste products, are excreted in the feces.

Food is mechanically chopped or ground by the teeth and lubricated by saliva and mucus secreted by the salivary glands. Some 1500 ml of saliva is produced per day. Saliva is mainly water but also contains amylase, an enzyme that begins to convert starch into sugars. The sensation of taste of dissolved substances is perceived by specialized nerve cells on the tongue. The slug (or bolus) of masticated food is forced into the pharynx and esophagus by the action of the tongue, elevation of the mandible (jawbone), hyoid, and thyroid cartilage, and compression of the cheeks. The epiglottis shields the larynx so that the food does not enter the airway. The food pellet is forced into the esophagus when the upper sphincter muscle relaxes and is then transported to the lower sphincter muscle and stomach by the peristaltic motion of the muscular esophagus, a tube about 25 cm long and less than 2.5 cm in diameter. The mucosa of the esophagus has an inner layer of stratified squamous epithelium. Glandular cells secrete mucus for lubrication, but no digestion occurs in the esophagus. The next layer is the lamina propria, with the mucularis mucosa on the outside, and mostly smooth (involuntary) muscle.

The stomach is a very muscular organ that mixes the food, expanding and contracting as the volume of its contents varies. The stomach lining has raised ridges, or rugae. The lining is of simple columnar epithelium, which lines the rest of the alimentary canal as well. Mucus-secreting cells of the epithelium dip into the lamina propria and form gastric pits, where gastric glands empty hydrochloric acid, the protein-digesting enzymes pepsin and renin, and lipase, which breaks down fats. The mucus protects the stomach from digesting itself. The stomach also secretes a factor that aids in absorption of vitamin B_{12}. A meal may remain in the stomach 1 to 4 hours, then pass through the pyloric sphincter into the small intestine (duodenum). Little absorption occurs in the stomach, except for alcohol and other readily soluble small molecules.

The small intestine is divided into the duodenum, the jejunum, and the ileum. It receives partially digested, liquid food (chyme) from the stomach through the pyloric sphincter and exits undigested and unabsorbed matter at the ileocecal valve into the cecum of the large intestine. Essentially all remaining digestion (aided by pancreatic juice and bile in the alkaline environment produced by intestinal secretions) and most of the absorption occurs in the small intestine. The duodenum is about 25 cm long, the jejunum 1.8 m long, and the ileum about 2.7 m long (about 5 m total length). The inner wall is characterized by circular folds and microscopic fingerlike projections (villi), giving the appearance of velvet, thus increasing the surface area. The lining is simple columnar epithelium backed by the muscularis mucosae, circular and longitudinal muscles that move food by peristaltic action, and serosa. Lymph vessels and nodes and patches of lymphoid tissue are distributed in the lamina propria. Nutrients are absorbed by capillaries and lymphatics in the villi and transported to the liver by the portal circulation or, indirectly, by the lymphatic system (lacteals, cisterna chylii, thoracic duct, venous system) to the liver. The small intestine and other organs in the abdominal cavity are supported by the ligaments and connective tissue of the mesentery, or omentum.

The large intestine (colon) is about 1.5 m long. It absorbs water and secretes mucus, but is basically a storage organ for feces.

The liver is the large gland (1.5 kg) located below the diaphragm in the upper part of the abdominal cavity. It has many functions. Of importance to digestion, it secrets about 500 to 1000 ml of bile a day, storing some 50 ml in the gallbladder, which empties along the common bile duct into the duodenum. Bile is 97 percent water, 1 percent bile pigments and salts, and 2 percent mineral salts and fatty acids. The bile salts, which are synthesized from cholesterol, aid in the digestion and absorption of fat by formation of a fine emulsion with water. The color of bile is yellow (produced by bilirubin) or greenish black (produced by biliverdin). These pigments are derived from hemoglobin. The liver also makes and stores vitamin A, makes heparin (an anticoagulant), fibrinogen, and prothrombin, breaks down RBCs and stores iron and copper, contains phagocytic cells (Kupffer cells), and removes many toxic substances from the blood.

The pancreas is a gland about 12.5 to 15 cm long located behind the stomach. It is a double gland, generating the pancreatic digestive juice, as well as the hormones insulin and glucagon from the pancreatic islands (islets of Langerhans). Some 2 liters per day of the pancreatic juice is secreted, an alkaline mixture of enzymes that participate in digestion of carbohydrates, proteins, and fats.

2.6 URINARY SYSTEM

The urinary system, illustrated in Fig. 2.9, is made up of the two kidneys, the ureters connecting the kidneys to the urinary bladder, the bladder, and the urethra, a canal leading from the bladder to outside the body. The function of the urinary system is to eliminate metabolic wastes and unnecessary chemicals, maintain acid-base equilibrium, and preserve the volume of body water. This involves exchanges between the blood plasma, fluid in the cavities of the kidney, and interstitial or extracellular fluid. Concentrated kidney fluid is urine.

The kidney is a bean-shaped dark red organ located in the retroperitoneal space (outside the peritoneum, or membrane covering other abdominal organs) in the posterior wall of the abdominal cavity at the level of the twelfth rib, embedded in protective fat. Each kidney is approximately 11.25 cm long, 5 to 7.5 cm wide, and 2.5 cm thick. The artery, vein, ureter, and nerves enter or leave at the hilus. The kidney is encapsulated in dense connective tissue. Internally, the kidney has a cortex and a medulla, made up of millions of tubules (nephron and collecting ducts), and a system of cavities (calyces joining into the renal pelvis) that collect the urine and conduct it to the ureter.

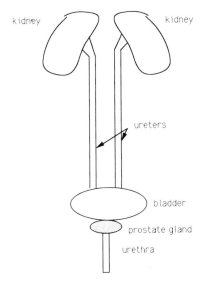

FIG. 2.9 Diagram of urinary system.

The functional unit is the nephron, as shown in Fig. 2.10. The renal artery branches several times, and eventually an afferent arteriole enters a glomerulus of capillaries. The blood leaves the glomerulus by an efferent arteriole. Some of the blood, less cells and large protein molecules, is filtered through thin porous layers of cells into the lumen, or capsular space, where the filtered plasma is collected by a proximal tubule at a rate of 125 ml per minute, per kidney. The driving force is the blood pressure (about 75 torr) less the counterpressure from the glomerular capsule (20 torr) and the protein osmotic pressure (30 torr) of the blood. The filtrate contains nitrogenous wastes (urea

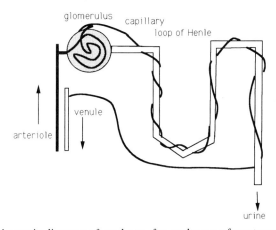

FIG. 2.10 Schematic diagram of nephron, for exchange of waste products and other compounds between blood and urine.

and uric acid) formed mainly in the liver, water, glucose, amino acids, and salts. The blood leaving the glomerulus by the efferent arteriole flows to a network of capillaries enveloping the tubules (loop of Henle) and collecting ducts, and thence to venules eventually returning to the renal vein at the hilus. About 99 percent of the filtrate is reabsorbed into the blood. Solutes such as glucose, amino acids, sodium, potassium, vitamins, and a small amount of protein are actively transported out of the tubule into the extracellular fluid and then reabsorbed in the capillary. Anions such as chloride and bicarbonate follow the cations out of the tubule. The removal of solutes increases the water concentration in the tubule, and osmosis of water occurs into the extracellular fluid and thence into the capillaries. Hydrogen and potassium ions and organic acids are transported in the opposite direction, from blood to extracellular space to inside the tubule. This helps maintain the blood pH. The final step is concentration of the urine by transporting water from tubule to extracellular fluid, under the influence of the antidiuretic hormone.

Urine flows out into the ureter, a fibromuscular tube about 28 to 35 cm long and varying from 1 to 10 mm in diameter. The ureter enters the bladder obliquely. Urine is propelled by peristaltic contractions. The bladder is a distensible storage vessel with a lining of transitional epithelium and a muscular wall. When filled to about 300 ml, there is an urge to urinate. The bladder is drained by the urethra, another fibroelastic, muscular tube some 4 cm long (female) or 20 cm long (male). Urination is under the voluntary control of sphincter muscles.

2.7 ENDOCRINE SYSTEM

The endocrine system comprises endocrine glands and specialized secretory cells in other organs, such as the islets of Langerhans in the pancreas, the mucosa of the stomach and duodenum, and certain cells in the kidney. The principal endocrine glands and some of the other organs involved are illustrated in Fig. 2.11. The products of the endocrine glands are *hormones*, chemicals released into the blood, where they are transported throughout the body and act on other glands and tissues. Some other substances are termed *parahormones* in that they have a similar effect. The parahormones, their sources, and principal functions are summarized in Table 2.4. The endocrine glands, hormones, and principal functions of hormones are given in Table 2.5. The endocrine system integrates the functions of the tissues and organs of the body, especially those having to do with metabolism; governs the development and growth of the body; controls development, growth, and regulation of the gonads and secondary sexual characteristics; regulates the internal environment (salt and sugar concentrations, rates of fat, protein, and sugar metabolism); and may affect emotions.

The "master gland" is the hypophysis, or pituitary, located under and

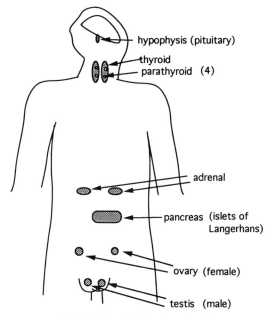

hypophysis (pituitary)
thyroid
parathyroid (4)
adrenal
pancreas (islets of Langerhans)
ovary (female)
testis (male)

FIG. 2.11 Endocrine glands.

connected to the hypothalamus of the brain. It is about the size of a pea and is divided into an anterior part (adenohypophysis) and a posterior part (neurohypophysis). The adenohypophysis, or glandular part, is provided with capillaries and cells that secrete several hormones, as listed in Table 2.5, that stimulate growth and development and regulate other endocrine glands (thyroid, adrenal cortex, and gonads). The neurohypophysis, or nervous part, does not secrete by itself, but stores hormones produced in the hypothalamus. It is supplied with nerves as well as capillaries.

The adrenal (suprarenal) glands, as the name suggests, are located above the kidneys. Each adrenal is a dual gland, with one set of hormones (epi-

TABLE 2.4 Parahormones

Parahormone	Source	Principal Functions
Carbon dioxide	Cell metabolism	Regulates respiration
Gastrin	Pyloric mucosa	Stimulates gastric juice secretion
Secretin	Duodenum mucosa	Stimulates pancreatic juice
Cholecystokinin	Duodenum mucosa	Stimulates release of bile by gallbladder
Enterogastrone	Duodenum mucosa	Inhibits gastric juice secretion
Histamine	Damaged tissues	Increases capillary permeability
Renin	Kidney	Stimulates vasoconstriction

TABLE 2.5   Endocrine Glands and Hormones

Gland	Hormone	Principal Functions
Hypothalamus	Oxytocin	Stimulates contraction of uterine muscle and release of milk by mammary glands.
	Vasopressin	Causes constriction of blood vessels and smooth muscle. Causes kidney to increase water reabsorption.
	Releasing factors	Regulate hormone secretion of anterior pituitary.
Hypophysis Anterior pituitary	Growth hormone	Stimulates development and growth
	Thyrotrophic hormone	Stimulates the thyroid gland
	Adrenocorticotrophic hormone (ACTH)	Stimulates adrenal cortex
	Follicle-stimulating hormone (FSH)	Stimulates growth of ovarian follicles and of seminiferous tubules of testis
	Luteinizing hormone (LH)	Stimulates the conversion of ovarian follicles into corpora lutea; stimulates secretion of sex hormones by ovaries and testes
	Prolactin	Stimulates mammary glands to secrete milk
	Melanocyte-stimulating hormone	Controls skin pigmentation in lower vertebrates
Adrenal (suprarenal) Medulla	Epinephrin (adrenalin)	1. Elevates blood pressure 2. Stimulates respiration 3. Slows digestive processes 4. Postpones skeletal muscle fatigure and increases muscle efficiency

TABLE 2.5 *(Continued)*

Gland	Hormone	Principal Functions
		5. Increases oxygen consumption and carbon dioxide production
	Norepinephrin	Raises blood pressure by stimulating contraction of muscular arteries
Cortex	Mineralocorticoids aldosterone	Regulates sodium-potassium metabolism (increases tubular transport of sodium; decreases transport of potassium)
	Glucocorticoids Cortisone Corticosterone Cortisol	Stimulate formation and storage of glycogen; help maintain normal blood sugar; maintain muscle strength; exert antiinflammatory effects; and increase resistance to stress.
	Cortical sex hormones Androgens	Exert antifeminine effects; accelerate maleness
	Estrogens	Exert feminine effects; accelerate femaleness
Thyroid	Thryroxin	Is main controller of catabolic metabolism
	Thyrocalcitonin	Prevents excessive rise in blood calcium
Parathyroid	Parathormone	Regulates calcium-phosphate metabolism
Pancreas (islets of Langerhans)	Insulin	Stimulates glycogen formation and storage; stimulates carbohydrate oxidation; inhibits formation of new glucose
	Glucagon	Stimulates conversion of glycogen into glucose
Thymus	Thymosin	Stimulates immunological competence in lymphoid tissue

TABLE 2.5   *(Continued)*

Gland	Hormone	Principal Functions
Ovary	Estrogen	Develops and maintains female secondary sexual characteristics; stimulates uterine lining to thicken
	Progesterone	Maintains female secondary sexual characteristics. Prepares uterus for reception of embryo; maintains pregnancy
	Relaxin	Relaxes pelvis and dilates cervix, aiding birth (Also derived from placenta)
Testis	Testosterone	Develops and maintains male secondary sexual characteristics

nephrin and norepinephrin) secreted by the inner part (medulla) and another set (steroids and sex hormones) secreted by the outer part (cortex).

The thyroid, located in the neck, is the largest endocrine gland, weighing 20 to 30 g. It has two lobes connected by an isthmus. The thyroid gland is made up of follicles of simple cuboidal or columnar epithelium with microvilli, on a layer of connective tissue, and infiltrated with blood and lymph capillaries and nerves. It secretes the hormone thyroxine, which is a compound with iodine. A deficiency of iodine in the diet can cause an enlarged thyroid, a condition known as goiter. Thyroxine is very important to metabolic control. The thyroid also secretes thyrocalcitonin, which helps control the concentration of calcium in the blood. The parathyroid glands are four bodies on the dorsal side of the thyroid lobes. Like the thyroid they are supplied with blood and lymph capillaries and nerves. They secrete a parahormone which regulates calcium metabolism.

The islets of Langerhans in the pancreas secrete insulin and glucagon, which control metabolism of glycogen (a starch) and glucose (a sugar). If a person's insulin production is insufficient, glucose is not metabolized properly, its blood concentration rises, and the individual suffers from hyperglycemia. Other disorders of glucose utilization result in diabetes mellitus.

The thymus is part of the lymphatic and immune system and is discussed in Section 2.9. The ovaries and testes are discussed in Section 2.10, Reproductive System.

2.8 NERVOUS SYSTEM

The functions of the nervous system include sensing the external and the internal environments, coordinating and controlling responses, and intelligence, or thought and memory. The CNS is composed of highly organized intercommunicating neurons in the brain and spinal cord. The peripheral nervous system (PNS), consisting of bundles of sensory and motor axons (nerves) and collections of cell bodies in the ganglia, extends throughout the body. A nerve may be sensory (afferent, sending information to the CNS) or motor (efferent, sending commands from the CNS to muscle or glandular cells). Subdivisions of the PNS and CNS are classified as voluntary or autonomic. Within the autonomic division, there is a set of sympathetic nerves and a set of parasympathetic nerves to the viscera, blood vessels, and glands. Afferent visceral nerves send sensations of sex, pain, nausea, hunger, and distension to the CNS. The special sense organs for vision (eye), hearing (ear), smell or olfaction, and taste are also part of the nervous system.

In the PNS, bundles of neuron axons are assembled into nerves, which also contain blood and lymph vessels, collagenous fibers, and an outer sheath of connective tissue for strength and support. Myelinated nerves are whitish and form "white matter." Cell bodies, dendrites, unmyelinated nerve fibers, and the supporting neuroglia cells are grayish and form "gray matter," found in ganglia. Gray matter (as well as white matter) is also found in the CNS, e.g., in regions of the spinal cord, and in the cerebral cortex of the brain. These regions are also supplied with blood, lymph vessels, and connective tissue. Neuroglia make up supporting tissue in the CNS. They include astrocytes, oligodendrocytes, and microgliocytes. Astrocytes are relatively large cells that contribute to repair, give support, and may transfer nutrients from blood vessels to neurons. Oligodendrocytes, which are smaller, participate in the formation and preservation of myelin sheaths. Microgliocytes are small cells and may be phagocytic, removing dead cells. Tumors often arise in the neuroglia.

Brain

The brain is shown in Fig. 2.12. It constitutes about 2 percent of body weight (about 1400 g in the adult male). It is located in the cranial cavity of the skull, enveloped in three membranes or meninges, and floats in cerebrospinal fluid (CSF). The meninges, from the outside in, are the tough fibrous *dura mater* attached to the skull, the thin but impermeable *arachnoid membrane* bathed in CSF, and the delicate vascular *pia mater* that supplies blood to the brain. CSF, which is similar to plasma, fills the ventricles and other cavities in the CNS, including the space between the spinal cord and the vertebrae.

The cerebrum is divided into left and right hemispheres, connected by nerve tracts to other parts of the brain. The tract connecting the two hemi-

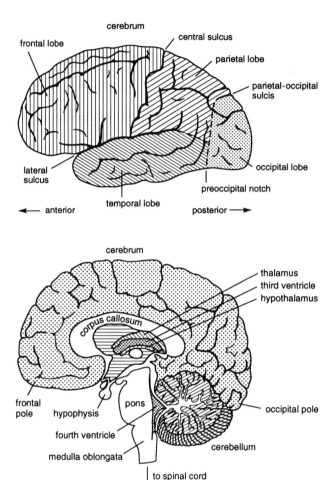

FIG. 2.12 Brain, showing lobes and sulci (fissures) and gyri (hills between sulci) of cerebrum; and section showing parts of brain.

spheres is the corpus callosum. The surface of the cerebrum is highly convoluted, thus increasing the area; the valleys are termed *sulci* or *fissures* (if deep), and the hills are called *gyri*. The outermost layer is the cerebral cortex (gray matter), and the myelinated nerves beneath constitute the cerebral medulla (white matter). The lateral sulcus (fissure of Sylvius) runs more or less horizontally from the front toward the back, whereas the central sulcus (fissure of Rolando) runs more or less vertically from the top toward the lateral sulcus. The central sulcus divides the frontal from the parietal lobe. The lateral sulcus divides the temporal lobe from the parietal and frontal lobes. The occipital lobe is situated posteriorly to the temporal lobe.

The thalamus is a processing center for sensory impulses traveling to the cerebrum, and for some motor functions. It is involved in sensations such as pain and touch and regulates the sleep-wake cycle. The hypothalamus is associated with many functions of the autonomic nervous system, communicates with the hypophysis, regulates water balance through a "thirst center," maintains heat balance and food intake, and is involved in emotional responses such as blushing and crying. The cerebellum regulates equilibrium, position sense, control of muscle tone, and overall coordination of muscular activity. The pons and medulla oblongata, and other structures mentioned, contain afferent and efferent nerve tracts and association neurons that modify or control reflexes and functions of the autonomic nervous system, including heart rate, respiration, and blood pressure through constriction of blood vessels.

There are 12 pairs of cranial nerves: I, olfactory (sense of smell); II, optic (sense of vision); III, oculomotor (to muscles controlling eyeball and pupil); IV, trochlear (additional eye muscles); V, trigeminal (sensory from face and motor to muscles of mastication, middle ear, and palate); VI, abducens (to an eye muscle); VII, facial (sensory from taste receptors, motor to nasal-oral cavity, lacrimal (tear) glands, salivary glands, facial and scalp muscles); VIII, vestibulocochlear (sound and equilibrium sensors in ear); IX, glossopharnygeal (sensory for part of the taste receptors, environs of tongue, blood pressure from the sensor in the carotid sinus, motor to the pharynx muscles and the salivary gland); X, vagus (sensory from the viscera and the upper respiratory tract, motor to some viscera, the pharynx, and the larynx); XI, accessory (larynx); and XII, hypoglossal (motor to muscles of the tongue).

Spinal Cord

The spinal cord is about 45 cm long and has an average diameter of 1 cm. It generally tapers to a point at the caudal end, but has notable cervical and lumbar enlargements. A cross section of the cord, showing also a simple spinal reflex arc, is seen in Fig. 2.13. There is a central X-shaped area of gray matter, surrounded by white matter. The anterior (ventral) surface is marked by a deep fissure. An afferent nerve fiber (axon) passes through a spinal ganglion of gray matter (enclosed, like the cord itself, in the meninges) and into the dorsal root of the spinal cord to synapse with one or more internucial

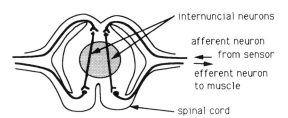

FIG. 2.13 Spinal cord and reflex arc.

or associative neurons that help to coordinate the response. Then a motor neuron axon leaves by the ventral root and travels to the effector, such as a skeletal muscle cell. An example of a simple reflex is the sensation of high temperature by a skin receptor, immediately followed by activation of a muscle to withdraw the body part from the hot object.

There are 31 pairs of spinal nerves (8 cervical, 12 thoracic, 5 lumbar, 5 sacral, and 1 coccygeal). Generally speaking, the nerves are associated with sensors and muscles at about the same level of the body, except for the lower limbs. There is also an autonomic division, which controls involuntary functions of visceral and other organs.

Eye

The eye is shown in Fig. 2.14. The eyeball (globe) is made up of a tough, fibrous, white outer layer (sclera) with a transparent curved window (cornea) in front. The rear of the eyeball is lined with a vascular, pigmented layer (choroid) that absorbs scattered light. The photosensitive layer (retina) lies on the choroid. The choroid thickens anteriorly to form the ciliary body (pigmented contractile tissue with smooth muscle fibers), which in turn acts on the suspensory ligaments of the elastic, transparent lens. The intensity of light reaching the retina is controlled by the diameter of the pupil, the opening in the iris. The chambers between the cornea and the iris, and between the iris and the lens, are filled with aqueous humor, similar to blood plasma without much protein. The chamber between the lens and the retina is filled with the transparent vitreous humor, a mucoprotein gel, that helps maintain the shape of the eyeball.

Light passes through a membrane and several layers of neurons before reaching the photosensitive rod and cone cells in the retina, and then the pigmented epithelium. Rod cells, which are some 200 times more numerous than cone cells except in the fovea centralis, are highly sensitive to light but do not signal color; rod vision is not as acute as cone vision. The cone cells

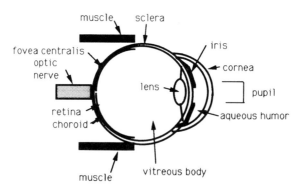

FIG. 2.14 Schematic diagram of eye.

are responsive to color, less sensitive to light intensity overall, but better for acute vision. Thus, best vision is achieved by orienting the eye and head so that the object of greatest interest is focused where the density of cone cells is maximum (and overlying cell layers are thinner), in the fovea centralis (at the center of the macula). There are no rod or cone cells in the optic disk, where the neurons converge to form the optic nerve. This is a blind spot but is usually not noticed.

The optic nerves cross and divide on their way to the visual centers in the brain. Thus the center in the left occipital lobe receives signals from the right side of the object as viewed by the left eye, and by the right eye; the right occipital lobe receives signals from the left side of the object as viewed by each eye (binocular vision).

The performance of the eye and brain as an optical measuring system can be analyzed in terms of (1) focus, (2) acuity or spatial resolution, (3) sensitivity and dynamic range, (4) color discrimination, and (5) binocular vision and depth cues.

Focus. The refraction at the cornea is fixed by its curvature and the differences in the index of refraction of the air (n = 1.000), the cornea (n = 1.376), and the aqueous humor (n = 1.336). The lens has a gradient index (n = 1.406 at the core, to 1.386 at the cortex), with aqueous humor on one side and vitreous humor (n = 1.337) on the other. The focal length of the cornea plus the lens is 17 mm, normally. The focal length of the lens, 64 mm, can be changed by changing its curvature. In the normal (emmetropic) eye, the image of an object at infinity is focused on the retina when the lens has its maximum curvature, which occurs when the ciliary muscle around the lens is relaxed. When the ciliary muscle contracts, the lens is flattened, its focal length is increased, and an object closer to the lens can be focused on the retina. This process is called *accommodation*. The closest point at which an object can be located and still be in focus is the near point, 25 cm in the average young adult. As a person ages, the lens usually becomes less elastic and the near point of accommodation gets larger, a condition termed *presbyopia* ("old sight").

A myopic (nearsighted) person is unable to focus a distant object on the retina, but can focus a near object. For an object at infinity, the focal point lies ahead of the retina. This condition can be corrected with a negative or diverging spectacle lens. Likewise, a hyperopic (farsighted) person can see distant but not near objects. Hyperopia can be corrected with a positive or converging lens in front of the eye. A third condition is astigmatism, which means that the focal point is different at different angles in the visual field. Astigmatism requires a correction with a section of a cylindrical lens, and this correction may be added to a correction for nearsightedness or farsightedness.

Acuity. Spatial and angular resolution are determined by size and spacing of the rods and cones in the retina, magnification, diffraction (as affected by pupil diameter), chromatic and other aberrations of the lens, and "image processing" within the retina and, presumably, in the brain. There are about 10^8 rods and 10^7 cones, distributed unevenly across the retina. The number of nerve fibers in the optic nerve is hundreds of times less than the number of rods and cones, thus some processing is done in the retinal neuron network and many rods at the periphery of the retina may be tied together. Most vision is restricted to a small area, the macula lutea (or yellow spot). Best resolution is achieved by aiming the eye so that the image falls within the fovea centralis in the macula, a region only 0.3 mm in diameter filled with cones and few, if any, rods. The image on the retina is small.

Diffraction depends on the size of the pupil, which may vary from a diameter of less than 3 mm in bright light to 8 mm in dim light. A typical pupil diameter is 3 to 4 mm. For a pupil diameter $D = 3.0$ mm and wavelength $\lambda = 555$ nm, the spread owing to diffraction is 4.5×10^{-4} radians. Actually, it has been found that aberrations rather than diffraction limit resolution, except for pupil diameters of less than about 1 mm, for which diffraction is limiting. The effect of aberrations can be investigated by measuring the modulation transfer function (MTF), or line spread function, as discussed by Williams and Becklund (see the Bibliography at the end of this chapter). Because of neuronal processing, however, the resolution as perceived is better than the resolution determined from physical measurements alone.

The resolution is usually determined by the subject's viewing eye charts from a fixed specified distance (i.e., a Snellen test with letters of progressively smaller size, Landolt C-rings of different diameters and orientations of the gap, bar charts, and displaced lines as in a Vernier caliper). These charts are black-on-white and thus have maximum luminance contrast. It is assumed that they are viewed with cone vision; therefore the background illuminance level or room lighting has to be sufficient for cones to be effective (at low light levels, only rods are sensitive enough). It has been found that visual acuity improves with increasing luminance. Vernier acuity, the ability to detect misalignment, is much better than acuity as measured by the ability to discern and thus tell the orientation of the gap in a C-ring (or to identify a letter). For the latter, the minimum detectable target angle subtended at the eye decreases from 10 minutes of arc at low background luminance to less than 0.5 minutes at high background luminance. A value of 1 minute of arc is typical for acuity.

Another aspect of acuity is the minimum luminance contrast that can be perceived for objects that have a range of gray levels or luminances instead of only black and white. This also depends on the background luminance level, as shown in Fig. 2.15. At low brightnesses, as in direct vision x-ray fluoroscopy, the eye cannot distinguish a target (e.g., the image of a tumor) unless it is at least 30 percent brighter or dimmer than the surrounding field.

Sensitivity. The eye can respond over a luminance range of 10^{10}:1. Only part of the adaptation, some 16:1, comes from the varying area of the pupil (8

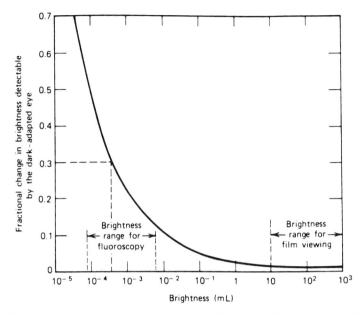

FIG. 2.15 Luminance contrast detectable as a function of background brightness. (Courtesy of Medical Physics Publishing Corp., Madison, Wis.)

mm diameter or f/2 in dim light to 2 mm diameter or f/8 in bright light). Furthermore, the iris takes about 5 seconds to close when coming from dark to bright surroundings and about 300 seconds to open fully when entering a dark area. Some of the dynamic range comes from the neural excitation range. However, most of the dynamic range is caused by the presence of the two kinds of receptors (rods and cones) and by changes in the visual pigment, rhodopsin. Rods are some 10^3 to 10^4 times more sensitive to light than are cones. They saturate at high levels of light, but when dark adapted, can detect just a few photons incident on the cornea. Rods are monochromatic; they do not distinguish colors, but the wavelength of maximum response is 510 nm, a blue-green. Cones can distinguish three primary colors (red, green, and blue) but are less sensitive than rods and do not increase sensitivity as much with dark adaptation. The wavelength of maximum responsivity is 555 nm (green). The cones adapt (increase sensitivity about 10 to 100 times) in 5 to 10 minutes. The cones adapt (increase sensitivity about 10,000 times) in about 30 minutes. These times presumably reflect the time it takes to increase the amount of rhodopsin in the cones or rods. The light-adapted predominantly cone vision is called photopic; dark-adapted, thus predominantly rod vision, is termed *scotopic*. Photopic vision is always assumed unless stated otherwise.

The transmission of the ocular media (cornea, aqueous humor, lens, vitreous humor, and overlying layers of the retina) varies with wavelength. In the green and red, the transmission is about 50 percent. Transmission decreases in the blue range, and ultraviolet is absorbed in the cornea. Transmission decreases and even less blue is transmitted (so that the lens appears yellow) with age and in the presence of some disease conditions. Cataract is an opacity of the lens, which may be caused by radiation. Blindness results unless the lens is removed. The usual visual spectrum is considered to extend from 400 nm (violet) to 700 nm (deep red), but at sufficiently high intensity and for some subjects, the response may extend to 750 nm or greater, and to less than 400 nm.

Color. The response spectra of the three kinds of cones are plotted in Fig. 2.16. Color blindness, which occurs when one or more of the receptors has reduced sensitivity, is found in 9 percent of males, and in 2 percent of females and is genetically linked. The most common form of color blindness is a weakness in perception of red. The human visual system can discriminate between thousands of colors by additive mixing of the three color receptors.

Depth Cues. Monocular vision provides cues or stimuli based on positions of objects (including overlap), apparent size of known objects (smaller at greater distance), linear perspective (convergence of parallel lines), aerial perspective (loss of contrast and detail because of atmospheric scattering and absorption), accommodation of focus, parallax (apparent direction and speed of objects when the viewer moves), contrast, and highlighting. Binocular vision adds the cues of convergence of the eyes (useful up to a few meters)

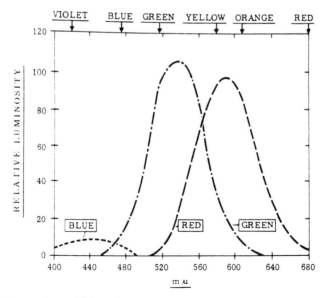

FIG. 2.16   Spectral sensitivity of the three types of cones. (Selkurt, E. E. 1966. *Physiology.* 2d ed. Boston: Little, Brown & Co.)

and steropsis, or binocular disparity (the image viewed with one eye is slightly different from the image viewed with the other eye).

Ear

The ear is shown in Fig. 2.17. Sound waves entering the external acoustic meatus vibrate the tympanic membrane (eardrum). The vibrations are transmitted by tiny bones (the malleus, the incus, and the stapes) to a membrane— the oval window, or fenestra vestibuli. This membrane in turn generates waves in the lymphlike fluid filling the semicircular canals and the cochlea. The cochlea is shaped like the tapering spiral shell of a snail. It is divided into two tubes, the scala vestibuli and the scala tympani. Waves propagate down the scala vestibuli to the tip of the cochlea and return up the scala tympani until they are damped by the round window (fenestra cochlea). Within the

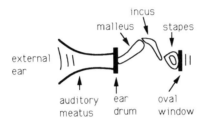

(a) Conversion of air vibration to vibration of oval window

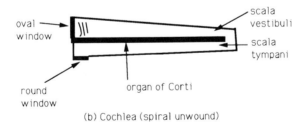

(b) Cochlea (spiral unwound)

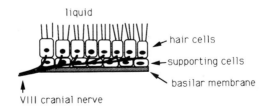

(c) hair cells in organ of Corti

FIG. 2.17   Ear: hearing organ. Semicircular canals are omitted.

cochlear duct is the organ of Corti, consisting of special hair cells and supporting cells on the basilar membrane. The hair cells convert mechanical energy into electrochemical energy and are connected to the cranial nerve VIII. The vestibular system is involved in maintaining equilibrium and sensing head movement. It includes the semicircular canals (oriented at right angles to each other), the semicircular ducts, the ampulla (or enlarged ends of canals containing crista), and the utricle (or saccule) in the vestibule. The ampulla contains nerve fibers, supporting cells, and hair cells with a sugar-protein mass on the hairs. Movement of the fluid during turning of the head sends out nerve impulses. The saccule and utricle are similar, with calcium salts in a gelatinous mass (otolith) on the hair cells.

The sense of hearing is able to respond to a wide range of sound intensities (10^{12}:1) over a frequency range of about 10 Hz to 20,000 Hz. The response of the auditory system is approximately logarithmic (in terms of perceived loudness as a function of intensity) and also depends on frequency. Greatest sensitivity is achieved at about 2 to 5 kHz. Intensity, the stimulus, is the sound power per unit area—W/cm^2 (equal to the square of the root mean square of the sound pressure). Sound intensity is measured in decibels:

$$N(\text{dB}) = 10 \log (I_1/I_2), \qquad (2.1)$$

where I_1 is the sound intensity of interest and I_2 is a reference intensity, usually taken as 10^{-16} W/cm^2. The relationship between the threshold of hearing and the intensity, as a function of frequency, for a young adult is plotted in Fig. 2.18. There is a decrease in sensitivity with age, at the higher frequencies. At about 140 dB, discomfort is felt more or less independently of frequency, and permanent damage and loss of hearing may occur for intensities of about 160 dB.

Loudness refers to the sensation of sound at intensities above threshold but below damage intensity. The unit of loudness is the phon, defined as the loudness corresponding to 1 dB intensity at 1000 Hz. For example, the loudness of a 10 dB sound at 1000 Hz is 10 phons, and so on. The ear is able to discriminate about 1 phon. At other frequencies, loudness is measured by adjusting the intensity until the loudness is perceived as loud as the known intensity of a 1000 Hz sound.

Smell and Taste

The senses of smell and taste depend on chemoreceptors to generate nerve impulses. The olfactory (smell) receptors are bipolar neurons located in the olfactory mucosa in the roof of the nasal cavity and connected rather directly to the brain. They sense substances dissolved in the mucus. The taste receptors are innervated epithelial cells located in pores in the taste buds on the tongue and oral cavity. The substances must be in solution. There are only four

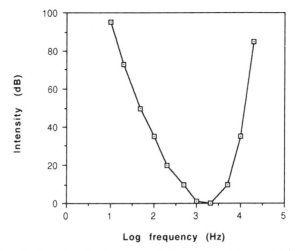

FIG. 2.18   Threshold of hearing in young adult (measured in decibels) as a function of frequency in hertz. Normal conversation (200–3000 Hz) corresponds to about 60 dB, heavy traffic to 80 dB, a symphony orchestra to 100 dB, and thunder to 100 dB. Threshold of feeling and discomfort is about 140 dB independent of frequency.

distinct tastes: sour, salt, sweet, and bitter. The "taste" of food is actually a combination of these tastes plus smell, texture, and temperature.

2.9   IMMUNE SYSTEM

The immune system defends the body against foreign substances, including microbes, viruses, and "non-self" cells (as in cancer and tissue transplants). It is also responsible for allergic reactions and for autoimmune diseases, in which the body's own cells are attacked. The AIDS virus attacks the T lymphocyte, reducing immunity and making the body susceptible to opportunistic infection. Because immunology is a complex subject and the target of intense current research, only its basic features are discussed here.

Figure 2.19 illustrates the main organs and cells of the immune system. The primary organs are the bone marrow and thymus, and the secondary organs are the blood and the spleen, lymph nodes, tonsils, and other lymphoid tissues. There are two kinds of immunity: humoral (antibodies produced by B lymphocytes from the bone marrow), and cell-mediated (T lymphocytes from cells produced in the bone marrow and then processed in the thymus). In addition, there are nonspecific killer cells, neutrophilic phagocytic polymorphonuclear leucocytes (PMNs) and macrophages (Mø's).

The bone marrow has been mentioned as part of the skeletal system and as the source of erythrocytes and leucocytes in the blood. Lymphoid tissues have been mentioned as parts of the lymphatic division of the circulatory

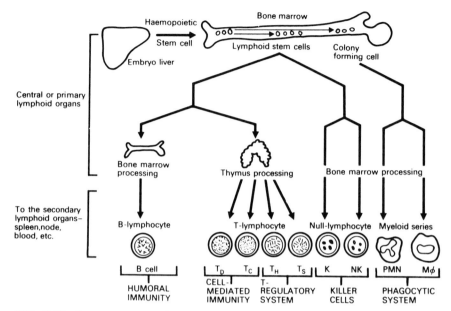

FIG. 2.19 Immune system. (From Bowry, T. R. 1984. *Immunology simplified.* 2d ed.: Oxford Univ. Press. By permission.)

system, and the thymus as an endocrine gland. The lymph nodes are distinguished by having afferent and efferent lymphatic vessels, whereas the others have arteries and veins and may have efferent lymphatic vessels. Lymphoid tissues are generally characterized by masses of lymphocytes and macrophages in follicles or corpuscles within a supporting reticular matrix, and expose the leucocytes to the circulating blood and lymph.

The body has a natural or inherent resistance to infection because of the PMNs and Mø's and the natural killer (NK) cells. PMNs mature in the bone marrow and are released into the blood, where they circulate for 6 to 7 hours and then migrate into tissues for 3 to 4 days. The monocytic Mø's (monocytes) circulate for 1 to 3 days and then migrate into tissues where they live for months. They are chemically attracted to sites of infection and arrive there in a few hours. These phagocytic cells also engulf and digest dead body cells and other debris. The NK cells are nonphagocytic and contribute to fighting viral infection with the help of a chemical, interferon.

Specific immunity against a certain cell or its clones depends on exposure to a genetically determined antigen on the cell membrane. An antigen is a foreign molecule (or, loosely, a cell or substance carrying the molecule) that stimulates an immune response and reacts specifically with the antibodies or sensitized T cells (T lymphocytes) produced. The active part of an antigen that reacts with an antibody is called an *antigenic determinant*, or *epitope*, and the antigen may have many epitopes of the same kind. The active immune response is diagrammed in Fig. 2.20. The antigen (Ag) is presented to small lymphocytes by an Mø. A small lymphocyte (called an immunocompetent cell) may have a specially shaped molecule on its membrane, a specific "antigen receptor" that fits and combines with, and thus recognizes, a specific antigenic determinant, X. There are some 10^{12} small lymphocytes in the body. In an unimmunized person there are some 10^8 different clones or populations, thus recognizing the same number of different antigenic determinants. Exposure of the body to a particular antigen stimulates the proliferation of one of the 10^8 clones (the one matching the antigen receptor on the small lymphocyte). This results in a relatively large population of B cells and cytotoxic T cells (T_C), and after modification of the antigenic determinant, a population of helper T cells (T_H) and delayed-hypersensitivity T cells (T_D). The immune reaction also leads to production of memory cells, which give a greater and more long-lasting response to a subsequent exposure to the antigen. The memory cells may last for years. This is the basis for immunization against infection.

A portion of the B lymphocytes transform into plasma cells that generate an antibody. An antibody is an immunoglobulin (protein). There are various

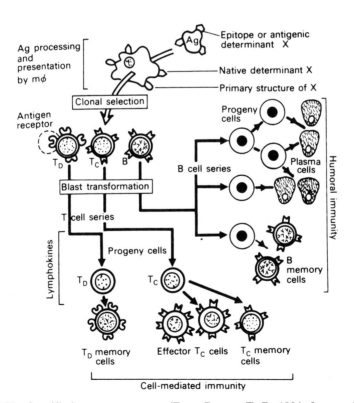

FIG. 2.20 Specific immune response. (From Bowry, T. R. 1984. *Immunology simplified*. 2d ed.: Oxford Univ. Press. By permission.)

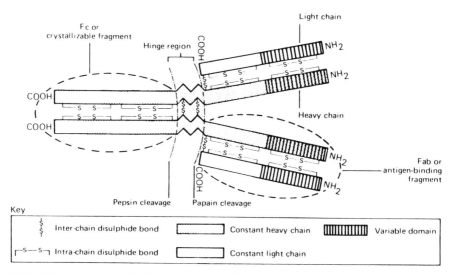

FIG. 2.21 Immunoglobulin B molecule. (From Bowry, R. R. 1984. *Immunology simplified*. 2d ed.: Oxford Univ. Press. By permission.)

kinds of antibody immunoglobulins (IgG, IgA, IgM, IgD, IgE). The Y-shaped structure of IgG is shown in Fig. 2.21. The number of antigen-binding sites per molecule varies from 2 to 10; IgG has two, one on each of the two legs. The ends of the legs are variable in composition and are able to bind to a specific antigenic determinant, e.g., on the surface of a bacterium. The bacterium is destroyed by a combination of the antibody and its complement, a system of many enzymes.

Cell-mediated immunity involves the thymus-derived lymphocytes, or T cells. This type of immunity is involved in tissue allograft rejection (e.g., in the case of organs donated by someone other than an identical twin, or in an incompatible blood transfusion), immune surveillance against cancer, delayed hypersensitivity or allergic reactions, and in resistance to intracellular infection, e.g., from viruses. The T_C lymphocyte attaches to the cell membrane at the antigenic determinant site and attacks the cell directly. The T_D lymphocyte involves chemical factors as well. The helper T cell, T_H, and the suppressor T cell, T_S, regulate the immune response. Helper cells activate the B and T_C cells, whereas suppressor T cells stop the immune response in order to prevent possible damage to "self" cells and to avoid exhaustion of the immune system when the antigen is no longer a threat.

2.10 REPRODUCTIVE SYSTEM

The male reproductive system is composed of testes, suspended within a sac of skin (the scrotum), ducts, and glands. Sperm is produced in the testis and collected and stored in the epididymis. Sperm is conducted through the ductus (vas) deferens to the ejaculatory duct and the urethra, which is shared with the urinary system. Nutrient-rich secretions of the prostate gland and the seminal vesicles are added, forming semen. Before ejaculation, the bulbourethral glands add secretions to lubricate the urethra. Sperm is then ejected into the vagina of the female. The testis is also an endocrine gland, producing the hormone testosterone, which is responsible for development and maintenance of the secondary male sexual characteristics and virility. Secretion of testosterone is controlled by a hormone produced by the anterior hypophysis.

The primary organs of the female reproductive system are the ovaries, which produce the ova and the hormones estrogen and progesterone, and the uterus. Estrogen is responsible for the development of secondary female sexual characteristics at puberty, sex drive, and stimulation of the uterine lining (endometrium) and the mammary glands. Secretion of female sex hormones is controlled by hormones from the hypothalamus and the anterior hypophysis. An ovum originates in a follicle in the ovary. A single ovum is released each month throughout the time between puberty and menopause. Following ovulation (rupture of a follicle), the follicle becomes the corpus luteum and secretes another female hormone, progesterone. This hormone is also involved in preparing the endometrium for childbearing. The ovum is collected in the uterine (fallopian) tube, where it may be fertilized, and then travels to the uterus. A fertilized ovum attaches itself to the endometrium (a process known as *implantation*).

Development of the fertilized ovum (zygote) to an embryo and then to a fetus occurs in the uterus, in amniotic fluid inside the amniotic membrane. The embryo or fetus is nourished through the placenta. The fetal blood is separate from the maternal blood, but oxygen and nutrients are transferred across the placenta from the maternal circulation to the fetal circulation. Some drugs and other chemicals will also cross the barrier, but others will not. At birth, the fetus is expelled, by muscular contractions of the uterine wall, through the vagina; the placenta and other contents are also expelled.

The breast (mammary gland) consists of exocrine glands and ducts imbedded as lobes in a fatty superficial fascia, together with nerves, blood, and lymphatic vessels, and covered with skin. The breast is supported by ligaments from the chest muscle and skin. The lymphatic vessels are important in that they drain fat from the milk and conduct infectious or malignant cells to the lymph nodes, especially in the axilla (armpit). The lactiferous (milk) ducts converge to openings in the nipple.

2.11 CANCER

Cancer is a neoplastic growth with uncontrolled proliferation of cells. It may occur in any of the organ systems, especially the bronchial mucosa (lung cancer), breast glandular tissue, colon and rectum, and urinary bladder. Proliferation may result either from uncontrolled division of cells (usually) or from an abnormally long lifetime of cells. In cancer, the usual controls such as "contact inhibition" that cause normal cells to stop dividing, do not function. A cancer may appear as a solid tumor or as proliferating cells in a liquid (in leukemia, an excess of WBCs; in ascites, individual cells in a body fluid other than blood).

Neoplasms may be benign or malignant. Some characteristics of each type are as follows:

Benign	Malignant
Usually grows slowly	Often grows rapidly
Grows expansively—no invasion or metastasis	Grows destructively—with invasion and metastasis
Retains mature, differentiated tissue	Composed of atypical tissue
Exhibits few mitoses	Exhibits many mitoses

Although a tumor or growth may be benign, it can still be dangerous simply because of its growth. For example, a tumor may grow into an airway, or pressure on the brain may result from a neuroma.

The induction of cancer is still not understood completely. However, some chemicals have been determined to be carcinogenic (e.g., benz(a)pyrene in tobacco smoke). Ionizing radiation may also induce cancer, particularly leukemia. Viruses have been implicated in at least a few animal tumors. In each case, the cancer is believed to start by a mutation in DNA of a single cell and the failure of the body's immune system to detect and eliminate the mutant cell. The carcinogenic process is believed to start when "oncogenes" are activated by the carcinogen.

Cancer, in general, is characterized by a latent period between induction of the transformation that triggers normal cells to continue dividing, and the actual detection of a tumor. Apparently, there is a period between the time when the cells have been modified and are ready to become a cancer, and the time actual proliferation begins. It is generally believed that two events and perhaps two carcinogenic agents are involved: an initial event (mutation or exposure to an "initiator") and a second event (or exposure to a "promoter").

Carcinoma in situ, shown in Fig. 2.22, is a condition in which an actual tumor has started to grow slowly but remains "in place" without invasion or metastasis. More rapid growth may depend on the tumor itself releasing a chemical (tumor angiogenesis factor) that promotes the growth of blood vessels to nourish the new growth. Thus solid tumors may range from a few cells to millimeter size (carcinoma in situ) to those several centimeters wide, limited by the ability of the host to sustain life. Tumors must be supplied with oxygen and nutrients, and waste products must be removed, hence they must be well

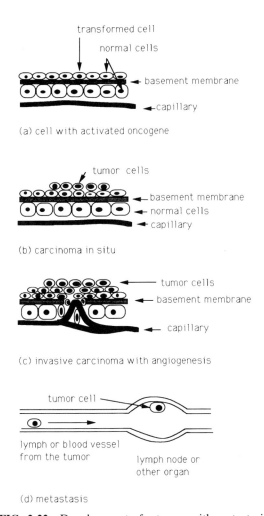

transformed cell

normal cells

basement membrane

capillary

(a) cell with activated oncogene

tumor cells

basement membrane

normal cells

capillary

(b) carcinoma in situ

tumor cells

basement membrane

capillary

(c) invasive carcinoma with angiogenesis

tumor cell

lymph or blood vessel
from the tumor

lymph node or
other organ

(d) metastasis

FIG. 2.22   Development of a tumor with metastasis.

supplied with blood vessels (or are supplied by diffusion from a nearby vessel, e.g., in carcinoma in situ).

Metastasis is the phenomenon of second tumors originating from cells that detach from the primary tumor, travel to a lymph node or other location in the lymph or blood, and grow there. Thus, even if the primary tumor can be treated, treatment is complicated by the secondary growths. The secondary growths or tumors retain the cellular characteristics of the primary growth. One may therefore speak of lung cancer or breast cancer (for example) outside the lung or breast, e.g., in the brain.

Solid tumors are characterized according to the type of tissue from which they originate: carcinoma (epithelial tissue), or sarcoma (connective and supporting tissue).

TABLE 2.6   Nomenclature of Solid Tumors

Tissue of Origin	Benign	Malignant
Epithelial		
Skin	Papilloma	Skin carcinoma
Glands	Adenoma	Adenocarcinoma
Liver	Liver adenoma	Hepatocarcinoma (hepatoma)
Pigment	Nevus	Malignant melanoma
Nerve	Glanglioneuroma	Neuroblastoma
Connective		
Connective	Fibroma	Fibrosarcoma
Cartilage	Chondroma	Chondrosarcoma
Bone	Osteoma	Osteogenic sarcoma
Muscle	Myoma	Myosarcoma

TABLE 2.7   Nomenclature of Leukemias

Cell Type	Origin	Leukemia	
Granulocytes	Bone marrow	Acute and chronic myeloid	(Myelosarcoma)
Lymphocytes	Lymphatic tissue	Chronic lymphatic	(Varying lymphomas, lymphosarcoma)

Cancer of nervous tissue is rare and has special names, such as *neuroblastoma*. A more detailed classification is given in Table 2.6. Leukemias are classified according to the type of cells involved, origin, and organ involved, as listed in Table 2.7.

BIBLIOGRAPHY

Bowry, T. R. 1984. *Immunology simplified*. Oxford: Oxford Univ. Press.

Cameron, J. R., and J. G. Skofronick. 1978. *Medical physics*. New York: John Wiley & Sons.

Crouch, F. E. 1978. *Functional human anatomy*, 3d ed., Philadelphia, Lea & Febiger.

Goss, C. M. 1973. *Gray's anatomy of the human body*. Philadelphia, Lea & Febiger.

Green, J. H. 1976. *An introduction to human physiology*. 4th ed. London: Oxford Univ. Press.

Kapit, W., and L. M. Elson. 1977. *The anatomy coloring book*. New York: Harper & Row.

Selkurt, E. E., ed. 1966. *Physiology*. 2d ed. Boston: Little, Brown and Co.

Suss, R., V. Kinzel, and J. D. Scribner. 1973. *Cancer: Experiments and concepts*. New York: Springer-Verlag.

Vander, A. J., J. H. Sherman, and D. S. Luciano. 1970. *Human physiology: The mechanisms of body function*. 4th ed. New York: McGraw-Hill.

Williams, C. S., and O. A. Becklund. 1972. *Optics: A short course for engineers and scientists*. New York: John Wiley & Sons.

CHAPTER 3

PHYSIOLOGICAL MEASUREMENTS

3.0 SENSORS, ELECTRONICS, AND DISPLAYS

Biomedical instruments, such as those used for measurements of physiological quantities, consist of a sensor (transducer, detector, gauge), signal processing (conditioning) electronics, and a display or output device. Actually, a few instruments still use mechanical devices for processing and display or recording, but these are being replaced by electronic versions. Optical processing is a possibility for the future, but there are as yet no true optical amplifiers or other convenient signal-processing devices in common use. Hydraulic, pneumatic, and magnetic devices do exist, but these are seldom used in biomedical engineering or medicine. Thus, biomedical sensors are usually transducers that convert the physical quantity of interest (temperature, pressure, etc.) into an electrical voltage or current signal.

Most sensors are analog, i.e., the amplitude of the electrical voltage or current varies continuously (and often proportionally) with the variation of the quantity to be measured, within certain operational limits. However, analog signals can be converted into digital equivalents by an analog-to-digital converter (ADC), and digital signals may be converted back to analog by a digital-to-analog converter (DAC). With digital signals, the information is contained either in the presence or absence of an output voltage pulse, the number of such pulses generated per second, or a train of logic pulses encoding a value in binary form (bits). Many nuclear particle and gamma-ray photon detectors are inherently digital, although the amplitude as well as the number of pulses (counts) per second is often significant.

There is already a well-developed technology for processing and analyzing electrical signals. Electrical analog signals can be amplified or attenuated, the frequency and time response modified, and signal waveforms analyzed by Fourier transform and other well-known methods. Pulse, count, or digital data can be analyzed for count rate and summed, can have background count rate subtracted, can be normalized and mathematically manipulated as numerical values, or considered as logic pulses. Digitized signals are used in many instruments, along with a microprocessor.

Display is used in the generic sense of an output device presenting data for human observation, automatic control, or computer processing. Common display devices include analog and digital meters, analog and digital recorders, oscilloscopes, computers with screens (monitors), and audio devices with variable pitch or loudness.

Mechanical measurands are involved in experiments, design, modeling, and clinical diagnosis and treatment of normal or pathological states of the skeletal and muscular systems, the circulatory system, the respiratory system, etc. Thermal measurands, temperature in particular, are of interest for a number of applications, such as diagnosis of infection and laser surgery. Measurements of optical quantities are associated with the eye and skin. Electrical measurements are important in the nervous and muscular systems (especially for the cardiac muscle). Chemical analysis is pertinent to evaluation of the circulatory and respiratory systems, as well as several others (e.g., the digestive, urinary, and endocrine systems). It is interesting to note that human beings sense and respond to mechanical displacement and forces, temperature, light, electricity, and chemicals, but not to electromagnetic waves outside the optical band nor to ionizing radiation (although cells may be damaged). The human body generates mechanical forces (muscle), heat (metabolism), electrical impulses (nerve, muscle), and many chemicals (digestive juices, hormones, etc.). Unlike some other organisms, it does not generate light (no bioluminescence) or other electromagnetic waves, strong electrical fields (as does the electric eel, for example), or ionizing radiation. However, electromagnetic and ionizing particle radiation are used for measurement, diagnosis, and therapy.

3.1 SENSORS FOR MECHANICAL QUANTITIES

Displacement may be measured for its own sake or, more frequently, as a measure of force or pressure displacing a mechanism such as a diaphragm or a spring. Common types of mechanical sensors are the resistive strain gauge, the resistive potentiometer, the inductive displacement transducer, the capacitive displacement transducer, the Hall effect transducer, the piezoelectric transducer, and the ultrasonic gauge (discussed in the Chapter 8, Diagnostic Ultrasound). A number of other sensors may also be employed; for a fuller description of all sensors of mechanical quantities, refer to the resources listed in the Bibliography at the end of this chapter.

Strain Gauge

A resistive strain gauge measures displacement by means of the change in resistance when the transducer element is strained (in tension, compression, or shear). Strain gauges can be used to measure force, given the conversion between force (or stress, force per unit area) and strain, i.e., Young's modulus. The resistive element may be a wire (typically 0.002 cm in diameter) or a semiconductor, and the gauge may be bonded or unbonded. A bonded gauge has the element cemented to a backing that is attached to the part where the strain is to be measured, as shown in Fig. 3.1. An unbonded gauge has the resistive element mounted between fixed and movable frames. If connected in a bridge circuit as shown, R_1 and R_4 increase when the moving

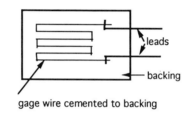

(a) bonded strain gage

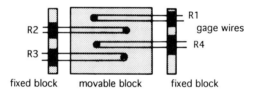

(b) unbonded strain gage

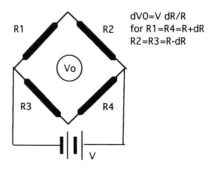

(c) Wheatstone bridge

FIG. 3.1   Strain gages and Wheatstone bridge.

member is displaced to the left, whereas R_2 and R_3 decrease, and the net change in voltage is doubled. All four resistances change the same amount with a change in temperature, and the temperature effect is canceled in the bridge. The allowable displacement is limited by the ultimate tensile strength and Young's modulus, and is small (tens of micrometers, perhaps). The force required is large, but strain gauges are really better suited for measurements of force than of displacement. Because the resistance change is often small and resistance also depends on temperature, temperature compensation is important.

The relationship between fractional resistance change and strain is called the gauge factor:

$$G = \frac{dR/R}{dL/L}. \tag{3.1}$$

The change in resistance comes about because of the changes in length and diameter and the "piezoresistive effect," in which the resistivity of the metal or semiconductor is changed. The gauge factor and the temperature coefficient of resistivity,

$$\alpha = \frac{(dR/R)}{(dT)}, \tag{3.2}$$

are given in Table 3.1 for some common materials. For metals, the gauge factor is relatively small (1 percent change in resistance is typical), linearity is better than 1 percent, temperature sensitivity is moderate, and the average resistance is 100 to 1000 Ω. The gauge factor for semiconductors may be 50 times larger, linearity is not very good, so that calibration is necessary, temperature sensitivity is relatively great, and the average resistance is 100 to 5000 Ω.

TABLE 3.1   Strain Gauge Factor and Temperature Coefficient

Material	G	$\alpha(\mathrm{K}^{-1})$
Advance	2.1	0.00002
Constantan	2.0	0.000002
Isoelastic	3.5	0.00047
Manganin	0.47	0.0000
Nichrome	2.5	0.0004
Nickel	12 to -20	0.006
Platinum	6.0	0.003
Silicon	120	0.006

Potentiometer

Another type of resistive device is the potentiometer, which converts either linear or angular (rotary) displacement into an output voltage by moving a sliding contact along a resistive element. The total resistance is R_L. An external voltage (V) must be applied across the resistive element. If the loading from the voltmeter is negligible, then the output voltage on the sliding contact is proportional to the displacement. The linear or angular resolution is limited by the wire diameter in wire-wound potentiometers. This problem is absent in potentiometers made with a cermet or conductive plastic. Other considerations in selecting a potentiometer are the moment of inertia and the starting and running force or torque. Other resistive devices include the elastic band, whose resistance varies with length. For measurement of an angle, the resistive potentiometer is often replaced by the digital shaft encoder, which generates pulses by means of optical or magnetic elements. The position or angle relative to a reference position or angle is determined by counting the number of pulses as the armature or shaft moves.

Inductive Displacement

Inductive transducers sense displacement by changing the self-inductance of a single coil or by changing the mutual inductance between two or more coils, usually by the displacement of a ferrite or iron core or plate. The self-inductance of a coil is

$$L = \mu N^2 \pi r^2 / l, \tag{3.3}$$

where μ is the permeability of the core material, N is the number of turns, r is the radius, and l is the length of the coil. The permeability of free space (and almost that of air) is $\mu_0 = 4\pi \times 10^{-7}$ henry/m.

The linear variable differential transformer (LVDT), a mutual inductance sensor, is often applied because of its good sensitivity (output per unit displacement), good linearity, and the relatively large displacement that can be handled. The LVDT (see Fig. 3.2) consists of a primary coil (P), excited by an AC current (typically 50 Hz to 20 kHz), with secondary coils S_1 and S_2 on each side. A ferromagnetic (ferrite) core or cylinder moves in the bore of the coil assembly. When the core is centered, equal voltages are induced in each coil, but they are connected in series opposition, so the net voltage out is zero. When the core moves toward S_1, the voltage in S_1 increases, the voltage in S_2 decreases, and the output voltage is in phase with the excitation voltage. When displaced toward S_2, the voltage across S_2 increases while the S_1 voltage decreases, and the output voltage is 180° out of phase with the excitation voltage. Circuits exist to detect the phase, so the direction of the displacement is measured as well as the amplitude. The amplitude of the output voltage is usually specified in terms of the sensitivity, e.g., 0.05 to 0.20 mV/μm dis-

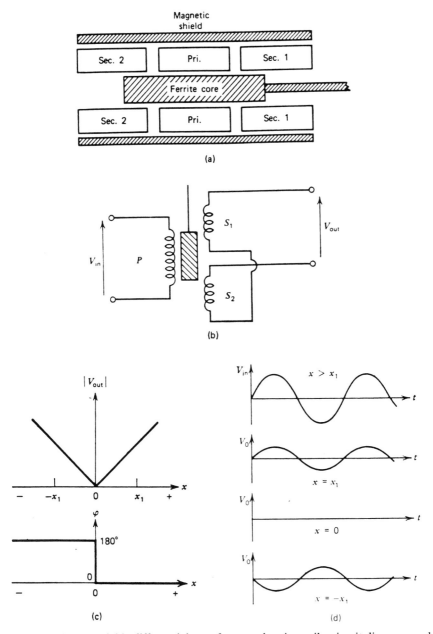

FIG. 3.2 Linear variable differential transformer, showing coils, circuit diagram, and input and output voltages as position of ferrite core is changed. (Cobbold, R. S. C. 1974. *Transducers for biomedical measurements.* New York: John Wiley & Sons.)

placement, per volt excitation. Typically, excitation is 1 to 10 V. LVDTs are available with full-scale displacements of 0.01 to 25 cm, linearity of 0.25 percent, and resolution of 1 μm or better. Core weight is 0.2 to 10 g, depending on the full-scale displacement.

A self-inductance device has been designed for intracardiac measurement of pressure by displacement of a mumetal core driven by a diaphragm. The coil is a variable inductor, determining the frequency of an oscillator. Demodulation of the frequency modulated signal gives an output approximately proportional to the pressure difference. The mass of the core and diaphragm are small, so the response to variations in pressure is good enough to sense heart sounds as well as the low-frequency blood pressure waveform. These are detected separately, with the use of low-pass and high-pass filters. Temperature compensation is achieved by a second coil with a nonmagnetic (Plexiglas) core.

Capacitive Displacement

The capacitance between two plane electrodes is given by

$$C = \frac{\varepsilon A}{d},$$ (3.4)

where ε is the permittivity of the dielectric between the plates (dielectric constant times permittivity of space, 8.85×10^{-14} F/cm), A is the area of an electrode, and d is the separation between them. When used as a pressure transducer or microphone, one electrode is a diaphragm. The fractional change in capacitance, dC/C, is proportional to the pressure and inversely proportional to the separation at zero gauge pressure. The simplest method of readout, adequate for a microphone, is to apply a DC voltage across the electrodes and amplify the AC signal generated by the vibrations of a diaphragm. The signal is small and drops to zero for very low frequency displacement (or slowly varying pressure).

Hall Effect

Figure 3.3 shows the elements of the Hall effect: the generation of a voltage across a thin film in which a current is passing at right angles to an applied magnetic field. The Hall voltage is expressed as

$$E = \frac{KIB}{t},$$ (3.5)

where K is the Hall constant for the material, I the current, B the magnetic flux density, and t the thickness of the film. Considering the thicknesses and currents that can be used without excessive heating, the output voltage is

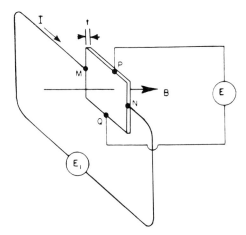

FIG. 3.3 Hall effect principle. Excitation voltage is E_1, current I, magnetic field B, slab thickness t, output voltage E.

usually in the range of tens of millivolts per tesla, using n-type germanium, indium antimonide, or indium arsenide. The Hall effect "chip" can be applied in different ways to measure displacement, e.g., moving the magnet or the chip in an inhomogeneous magnetic field, or a ferromagnetic part in the magnetic circuit (for changing the air gap, for example). With AC excitation of the current, a voltage will also be induced in the loop formed by the chip and its leads. It may be desirable to cancel this transformer voltage by connecting another single-turn coil in series opposition.

Piezoelectric Effect

When an asymmetrical crystal such as quartz is deformed, a charge is generated on the surface. The strain is typically very small, about a micrometer, so the piezoelectric transducer is best suited for measuring force or pressure. The relationship between charge Q and force F is

$$Q = DF, \tag{3.6}$$

where D is the piezoelectric coefficient listed in Table 3.2. A change in charge

TABLE 3.2 **Piezoelectric and Dielectric Constants**

Material	D (pC/N)	Dielectric constant	Maximum stress (MN/m^2)
Quartz	2.3	4.5	98
Barium titanate	140	1200	80
Lead niobate	200	1500	20

can be measured by a charge-sensitive amplifier, or the change in voltage across the crystal measured, where

$$V = Q/C \tag{3.7}$$

and the capacitance C is given by equation 3.4. The dielectric constants for the piezoelectric materials are also given in Table 3.2. Because of charge leakage, the piezoelectric transducer is not suitable for static or low-frequency measurements, and there is a mechanical resonance at some higher frequency (exploited in crystal-controlled oscillators).

A piezoelectric transducer can also be used to reverse, changing its thickness, volume, or shear when an external voltage is applied across the piezoelectric element. Such devices are often used to generate ultrasonic waves or pulses.

3.2   SENSORS FOR PRESSURE, FLOW, AND VOLUME

Sensors for measurement of fluid pressure, flow rate or fluid velocity, and volume are discussed in this section. In biomedical engineering and clinical practice, measurements of blood pressure and flow rate or output are of special interest. One may also wish to measure or monitor intracranial pressure or intraocular pressure, the flow of other body fluids, and the volume of air in the lungs.

Direct Pressure Gauge

Pressure is defined as force per unit area. Several sensors suitable for measurement of force are discussed in Section 3.1. Application of these and other transducers for sensing fluid pressure are discussed in this section. Figure 3.4 shows a system for direct measurement and monitoring of blood pressure. The pressure transducer itself is a strain gauge coupled to a diaphragm. The blood or other fluid is contained in a clear plastic chamber to allow checking for air bubbles, and a side port permits flushing the dome to keep clear the catheter (a hollow, small-diameter tube). An intravenous drip of heparinized normal saline or 5 percent dextrose in water, commonly employed as the fluid column, helps to maintain patency (openness) of the artery or vein and to prevent blood clots. The catheter may be inserted into a blood vessel for measurements at various locations. The infusion manifold allows blood samples to be withdrawn, and the monitor displays the pressure wave. It usually computes and displays the systolic (maximum) and diastolic (minimum) pressures, as well as the heart rate (beats per minute). A record of blood pressures in the heart and aorta is plotted in Fig. 3.5, which also plots heart sounds and the electrocardiogram (discussed in a later section).

In any measurement of fluid pressure, one has to consider the fluid "head"

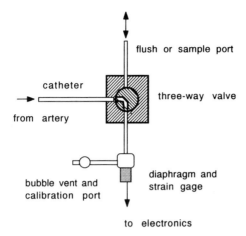

FIG. 3.4 Direct measurement of blood pressure. Interarterial catheter may be flushed with heparin to suppress clotting.

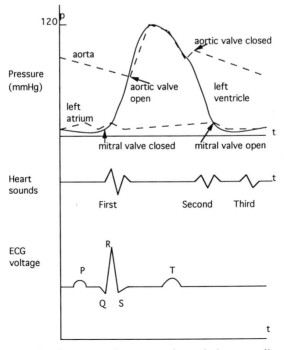

FIG. 3.5 Blood pressure, heart sounds, and electrocardiogram.

owing to gravity and the dynamic effect if the fluid is flowing. The total fluid energy per unit volume is expressed as

$$E = P_s + \rho gh + \rho v^2/2, \tag{3.8}$$

where P_s is the static pressure or energy (energy required to move 1 cm³ of fluid against the static pressure without imparting any velocity to it), the second term is the gravitational potential energy, and the third term is the kinetic energy of the fluid in 1 cm³, ρ is the density, g is the acceleration resulting from gravity, h is the height of a fluid column above an arbitrary reference level, and v is the fluid flow velocity. If there is no friction, E is constant, but one kind of energy may be transformed into another. When a tube connected to a pressure gauge is inserted in the fluid stream and faces upstream, the pressure measured is static plus kinetic. If the tube opens at right angles to the flow, static pressure is measured. The kinetic energy contribution may be significant in measurement of blood pressure, where flow velocities may be 10 to 100 cm/s. The effect of gravitational potential is canceled by locating the tube opening at the reference level (e.g., the level of the heart).

Indirect Pressure Gauge

A more convenient, noninvasive gauge is desired for routine measurements of blood pressure. The familiar sphygmomanometer, or an automated version of it, is used to obtain an average arterial pressure. An inflatable cuff with an attached manometer (mercury column or aneroid pressure gauge) is placed around the subject's upper arm in order to collapse the brachial artery when the cuff is inflated to above the maximum (systolic) pressure. A stethoscope or microphone is placed over the artery distal to the cuff, and the operator listens for the Korotkoff sounds generated by the restricted blood flow, as the cuff pressure is lowered gradually to the lowest (diastolic) pressure. The sounds and applied pressure are correlated as shown in Fig. 3.6. A similar method can be used on the artery in a finger, with detection of the volume change effected with a Light Emitting Diode source and a photodiode detector as the cuff pressure is cycled.

Electromagnetic Flow Meter

Blood and other body liquids are electrically conductive. When a conductor is moved perpendicularly to an applied magnetic field, a voltage or emf E is generated that is at right angles to both the flow vector and the magnetic field vector (dynamo effect), as illustrated in Fig. 3.7. The emf is

$$E = 2aBv = 2BQ/\pi\, a, \tag{3.9}$$

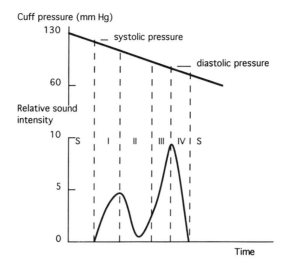

FIG. 3.6   Principle of indirect blood pressure measurement with sphygmomanometer. S = silence, Phase I: snapping tones, Phase II: murmurs, Phase III: thumping, Phase IV: muffling.

where a is the radius of the conductor, B the magnetic flux density, v the average fluid velocity, and Q the volumetric flow rate. The emf is measured across electrodes contacting the vessel wall through an electrolyte. With a blood vessel radius of 0.1 cm, flow rate of 1 cm^3/s, and $B = 300$ gauss, V is on the order of several microvolts. The magnetic field may be pulsed or modulated, thereby modulating the emf and reducing the problem of DC polarization of the electrodes, but introducing a "transformer" emf that has to be canceled. The sensor is usually a "clip-on" probe that can be opened to accommodate the blood vessel and then closed to complete the magnetic field. The internal diameter of the probe is selected to make good contact between the electrodes and the vessel wall. The Bibliography at the end of this chapter should be consulted for books giving more details on the design and use of electromagnetic flow meters, as there are a number of corrections necessary to obtain accurate measurements.

Transit Time Flow Meter

The average fluid velocity (v) can be derived from the difference in time for an ultrasonic pulse to travel upstream and downstream between two fixed points (the phase shift in a cw measurement may be used instead of pulse transit time). In Fig. 3.8, consider the transit time between ultrasonic transducers. A and B, separated by distance D and oriented at angle θ to the flow

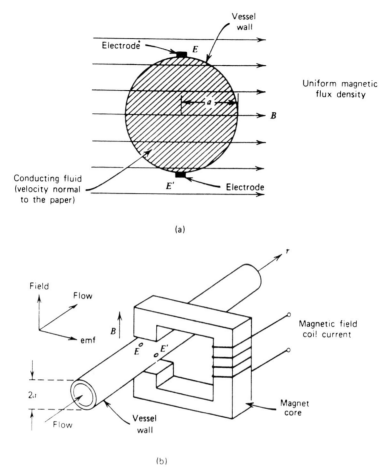

(a)

(b)

FIG. 3.7 Principle of electromagnetic flowmeter. (Cobbold, R. S. C. 1974. *Transducers for biomedical measurements*. New York: John Wiley & Sons.)

axis. The component of the average fluid velocity along the line joining A and B is $v \cos \theta$. Then the transit time traveling upstream is

$$t_u = \frac{D}{c + v \cos \theta} \tag{3.10a}$$

and traveling downstream (pulses from B to A)

$$t_d = \frac{D}{c - v \cos \theta}; \tag{3.10b}$$

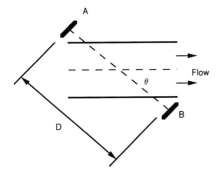

(*a*) Ultrasonic transducers *A* and *B*, separated
by distance *D* and located at angle θ to flow axis,
transmit and detect pulses. Transit times vary
with velocity of fluid.

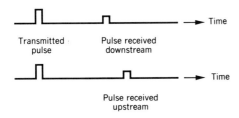

Transmitted
pulse

Pulse received
downstream

Pulse received
upstream

(*b*) Transmitted and received pulses.

FIG. 3.8   Principle of transit time flow
meter.

hence,

$$\Delta t = \frac{2Dv \cos \theta}{c^2} \qquad (3.11)$$

approximately, where c is the velocity of sound in the fluid, 1.5×10^5 cm/s
in blood. Quite small time differences have to be measured, because v is
much less than c.

The Doppler shift in frequency of a reflected (scattered) ultrasound wave
can be used to measure the average flow velocity and, hence, the volumetric
flow rate if the vessel diameter is known. In blood, the scattering is produced
by the blood cells, principally erythrocytes. The difference in speed going
upstream and downstream results in a change in frequency by the Doppler
effect, and the greater the velocity of the erythrocytes, the greater the frequency shift. The Doppler shift is discussed in more detail in Chapter 8,
Diagnostic Ultrasound.

Tracer Dilution Flow Meter

The average flow rate can be measured by mixing a very small amount of tracer or indicator with the fluid. Fick's principle states that if the concentration of the tracer is known at the input and output of an organ (for example), as well as the amount of tracer added to or eliminated from the organ per unit time, then in the steady state the volumetric flow rate is

$$Q = A/(c_i - c_o), \tag{3.12}$$

where A is the amount of tracer removed or added per second, c_i is the tracer concentration at the input, and c_o the concentration at the output. The tracer may be an optical dye whose concentration is measured photometrically, a radioactive material in soluble form whose relative concentration is measured by a nuclear detector, a radiopaque contrast agent measured by x-ray transmission, or any chemical substance that can be analyzed on-line or by sampling. A known amount of tracer is added, and the concentrations are measured before and after the injection point. A problem in measuring blood flow rate by Fick's principle is recirculation of the tracer, unless the tracer is eliminated somewhere in the circuit.

Another approach is rapid injection of an amount (I) of the tracer, and measurement of the output concentration as a function of time, $c(t)$, the so-called indicator dilution curve shown in Fig. 3.9. Assuming all of the tracer is transported to the output,

$$dI = Qc(t), \tag{3.13}$$

and the flow rate Q is equal to I divided by the integral of $c(t)$ from zero to infinity, after extrapolating into the times where recirculation modifies the dilution curve.

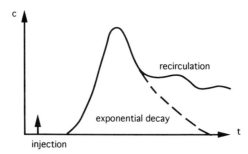

FIG. 3.9   Tracer dilution curve, concentration (c) vs time (t) with and without recirculation, for rapid injection.

Other Flow Meters

Standard flow meters, such as those using a signal-generating turbine in the stream or measurement of pressure drop across an orifice, may be used for physiological measurements.

Plethysmograph

A volume-measuring device is called a *plethysmograph*. A common type is the spirometer for measuring lung capacity. It consists of a lightweight bellows with some kind of readout. One can also measure volume by integrating the flow as measured with a pneumotachograph transducer. The record of a typical lung function test is shown in Fig. 3.10. The tidal volume (TV) is the volume of air inspired or expired in each normal, resting respiratory cycle. The inspiratory reserve volume (IRV) is the additional volume of air that can be inspired with maximal effort. The expiratory reserve volume (ERV) is the additional volume that can be expired with maximal effort, leaving the residual volume (RV) in the lungs. The vital capacity (VC), measured as a function of time, is the volume of air that can be expired with maximal effort after inspiring with maximum effort. It is equal to the sum of TV, IRV, and ERV. Total lung capacity (TLC) is equal to VC plus RV. The functional residual capacity (FRC) is the sum of RV and ERV, and is often used as a reference volume.

A mechanical model of the respiratory system is shown in Fig. 3.11. Compliance (C) (represented by a spring) is an important characteristics; it is the ratio of the change in volume (dV) for a given change in pressure (dp). It corresponds to the elasticity of the chest wall and diaphragm. In normal adults

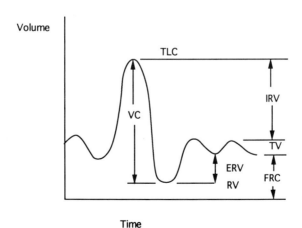

FIG. 3.10 Measurement of lung volume. *TV* = tidal volume, *IRV* = inspiratory reserve volume, *ERV* = expiratory reserve volume, *RV* = reserve volume, *VC* = vital capacity, *TLC* = total lung capacity, *FRC* = functional reserve capacity.

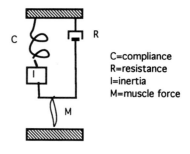

(a) Mechanical model of respiratory system

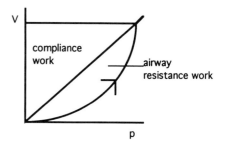

FIG. 3.11 Model of respiratory system.   (b) p-V and work diagram

the compliance is 0.18 to 0.27 l per cm H_2O pressure change. A stiff, fibrotic lung has a lower compliance, whereas in emphysema, the compliance is greater. Another characteristic is airway resistance (R) (represented by a dashpot), the ratio of the pressure drop along the airway to the flow rate. An average value for an adult is 3.3 cm H_2O pressure drop for 1 l/sec flow rate. The resistance increases in obstructive diseases such as asthma or emphysema. Also represented in the model is the inertia (I) of the moving parts and the muscle force (M). When the lungs are unable to oxygenate the blood sufficiently, a mechanical ventilator may be used to pump air or oxygen into the lungs.

3.3 TEMPERATURE SENSORS

There is no sensor for heat energy as such. Inferences about heat transfer are made from measurements of temperature changes on adding or removing heat, knowing the heat capacity; from the mass of material changing phase (freezing or melting, condensation or vaporization), knowing the latent heat;

or from the electromagnetic energy radiated, knowing the emissivity of the surface and measuring the spectrum or equivalent temperature of a blackbody radiator.

The human body has a system for regulating temperature within a small range, balancing heat losses (primarily by air convection and evaporation of sweat from the skin) against heat gains from metabolism and exercise. The basal metabolic rate (energy consumption while at rest) in an adult male is about 120 W (120 J/s), corresponding to a useful food intake of 2478 kilocalories per day (about 2500 C/day). The body attempts to maintain a constant core temperature. Measured orally (under the tongue), the normal temperature is 37°C (98.6°F, 310 K). Rectal temperature is about 0.5°C higher. Body temperature varies with time of day and exercise, but a temperature consistently elevated or depressed—by more than 1°C—is a sign of disease, such as in infection. Thus, physiological thermometers should be capable of measuring temperatures a few degrees on either side of 37°C, with an accuracy 0.5°C or better. Higher local temperatures are encountered in hyperthermia and in laser surgery.

Thermoresistive Thermometer

Metals and semiconductors change their resistance with changes in temperature. For most metals, the resistance increase is positive, whereas semiconductors may be formulated to have either a positive or negative coefficient. For small temperature changes

$$R = R_O\{1 + \alpha(T - T_O)\} \tag{3.14}$$

where R_O is the resistance at the reference temperature T_O. The temperature coefficient (α) and the resistivity at room temperature (25°C) are given in Table 3.3.

The platinum resistance thermometer is stable and linear (0.2 percent) and capable of accuracy within 0.001°C. It is often used as a reference standard,

TABLE 3.3   Temperature Coefficient and Resistivity

Material	$\alpha(°C^{-1})$	ρ (Ω-cm)
Copper, annealed	+0.0039	1.7×10^{-6}
Nichrome	+0.0004	1.0×10^{-4}
Mercury	+0.0009	9.8×10^{-5}
Platinum	+0.0038	1.0×10^{-5}
Carbon	−0.0005	3.5×10^{-3}
Silicon (doped)	+0.007	1.4 (p-type)
	+0.6	(n-type)
Thermistor	−0.04	1000 (metal oxide)
	+0.10	(titanates)

although the temperature coefficient is small. Sources of error include changes in electrical lead resistance, thermal emf's generated at contacts, and self-heating. The resistance is best measured in a null bridge circuit with three identical leads (usually copper) running to the thermoresistive element. The leads all experience the same temperature variation, and the bridge cancels the contribution of the lead resistance. Thermal emf's can be minimized by arranging that all contacts be at the same temperature or by using AC excitation, preferably with a phase-sensitive null detection circuit. Self-heating by the current through the resistive element can be made negligible by decreasing the supply voltage to about 50 mV and increasing the null amplifier gain to compensate. When less accurate measurements are adequate, a deflection-type bridge circuit and just two leads may suffice.

Thermistors (thermally sensitive resistors) are frequently used for physiological or clinical measurements because their temperature coefficients are much larger than those of metals, and the thermistor bead can be very small (thus, speed of response to a temperature change can be very good—within milliseconds). Signal conditioning and readout circuits for the positive temperature coefficient materials (silicon doped to about 10^{16} atoms per cubic centimeter, and strontium/barium-titanate–type thermistors) are designed in much the same way as for metallic thermoresistive elements. The negative temperature coefficient devices are, however, very nonlinear at higher currents because of self-heating. It is even possible for the thermistor to "run away" and be destroyed unless current is limited by another element, because increased power dissipation results in lower resistance and more heating. Figure 3.12 illustrates a linearized temperature-measuring circuit and examples of thermistor probes (a glass-protected bead and a bead mounted in a hypodermic needle). The voltage applied to the thermistor R_T is 50 mV. Current feedback in an operational amplifier creates a virtual ground at the input of the amplifier and allows the current through the thermistor to be measured without affecting the voltage across it. With a high amplifier input impedance, the current through feedback resistance (R_F) equals the thermistor current less the offset current (i_o), and the output voltage is linearly related to the thermistor current and, thus, to the temperature.

Thermoelectric Thermometers

A current flows when two dissimilar metals are connected in a closed circuit and the junctions are at different absolute temperatures, T_1 and T_2 (see Seebeck effect). If the circuit is opened, a voltage or emf can be measured:

$$V = \beta(T_1 - T_2) + \gamma(T_1^2 - T_2^2). \qquad (3.15)$$

Over a limited temperature range, the quadratic dependence is not too large,

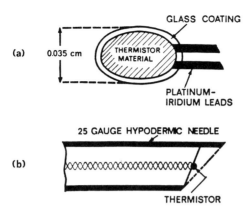

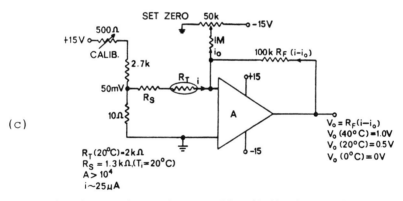

FIG. 3.12   Thermistors and operational amplifier. (Cobbold, R. S. C. 1974. *Transducers for biomedical measurements*. New York: John Wiley & Sons.)

and one can write for the differential coefficient for the thermocouple, the thermoelectric power or sensitivity,

$$S = \frac{dV}{dT_1} = b + 2\gamma T_1 \tag{3.16}$$

The sensitivity at 20°C for some common thermocouples is listed in Table 3.4, together with an assessment of potential accuracy. Because a thermocouple responds to the difference in temperature between the hot junction and the cold junction, it is necessary either to hold the cold junction to the reference temperature (0°C) by immersing the cold junction in an ice bath,

TABLE 3.4   Thermocouple Sensitivity and Accuracy

Thermocouple	Sensitivity $\frac{\mu V}{°C}$	Accuracy
Copper/constantan	45	+/−0.5%
Iron/constantan	52	+/−1%
Chromel/alumel	40	+/−0.5%
Chromel/constantan	80	
Platinum/platinum-rhodium	6.5	+/−1%

or to compensate for changes in temperature of the cold junction by an electronic circuit (possible over a range of several degrees C). Such a circuit generates an emf that varies with temperature and nullifies the emf from the varying cold junction temperature. The thermal emf from the measuring thermocouple may be measured with a digital voltmeter or with a self-balancing (servo-controlled) potentiometer. Thermocouples can be formed by spot welding two dissimilar metal wires and can be made as small as thermistors and incorporated in a probe, hypodermic needle, or small-diameter catheter.

3.4   SENSORS FOR BIOELECTRIC POTENTIALS

Bioelectric potentials are action potentials of muscle and nerve cells and may be sensed by appropriate electrodes. Electrodes placed on the skin or inserted as needles through the skin are responsive to the currents from many cells; these are used in electromyography, electrocardiography, and electroencephalography. Electrical impulses generated by light incident on the retina can be sensed by an electrode on the cornea or across the retina (electroretinography). In some cases, e.g., during surgery, the electrode is placed directly on the organ. These are all varieties of what may be termed *macroelectrodes*. Potentials associated with individual cells are measured by *microelectrodes*, with tips smaller than a cell to minimize the disturbance on penetrating the cell membrane. Macroelectrodes are designed to make a reasonably low impedance contact with the skin or an organ. In all cases, potentials are measured with respect to a reference electrode at some relatively inactive site on the body.

Macroelectrodes

Electrodes for biopotentials induced at the skin may use a metal-electrolyte connection (direct-contact type) or may be capacitively coupled. The direct-contact type is a transducer from ion transport in an electrolyte, such as the conducting tissue fluids, to electron transport in a metallic conductor. The capacitive-coupled type transduces ion currents into a displacement current in the capacitor plate.

The direct-contact type connection on the skin surface is designed to overcome the high impedance (resistance) of the stratum corneum, or horny layer of the epidermis. It may consist of a metal such as silver or stainless steel, with a paste or jelly electrolyte (containing chloride and other ions). The recessed electrode shown in Fig. 3.13 is becoming more popular than flat or suction cup electrodes because it produces fewer artifacts resulting from patient movement. The electrode area is about 1 cm^2 and the resistivity of the paste is typically 5 to 400 Ω-cm, which, for a 1-mm-thick layer gives an impedance of 40 Ω or less. Another approach is to penetrate the stratum corneum with thousands of fine points. Resistivity is about the same as for flat electrodes with electrolyte paste. Even plain metal (e.g., stainless steel) electrodes can be applied without paste; the impedance is high (a few megohms), but they are usable with proper electrostatic shielding against interference and a high impedance amplifier. A shielded FET preamplifier can be mounted at the electrode, for example. Another type of direct-contact electrode consists of an insulated wire or needle with an uninsulated end, inserted transcutaneously or directly into an organ, bypassing the skin impedance.

Capacitively coupled electrodes may contact the skin in order to maintain electrode-skin spacing, but they measure the displacement current induced by AC waveforms, rather than charge transport. The electrode may be made of tantalum (anodized to form an insulating coating, thus capacitor dielectric), a doped silicon semiconductor with silicon oxide dielectric, or metallized dielectrics such as barium titanate. The idea is to make the dielectric as thin as possible and of high dielectric constant, so as to increase the capacitance.

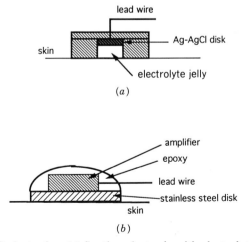

FIG. 3.13 ECG electrodes: **(a)** floating electrode with electrolyte jelly; **(b)** dry electrode with very high impedance amplifier.

Electrode area is usually about 1 cm^2, capacitance a few thousand picofarads, and DC insulation resistance a few thousand megohms.

Microelectrodes

When the potential across a single cell is to be measured, the measuring electrode may be made of metal drawn to a fine tip and insulated except at the very end. Another design uses a glass tube with a fine tip about 1 μm in diameter, with an Ag-AgCl electrode in the stem and filled with KCl electrolyte. The impedance of microelectrodes and macroelectrodes varies with frequency. The impedance (reactance and resistance) can be measured for precise work involving high fidelity reproduction of the bioelectric potential waveforms. The intracellular potential is about 50 to 100 mV. The action potential of nerves propagates with times on the order of milliseconds. Muscle cells propagate the action potential much more slowly.

Electromyography

An electromyogram (EMG) generally measures the bipotential waveform from many skeletal muscle fibers or motor units (a branching motor axon and 25 to 200 muscle fibers). It may be obtained with a concentric needle electrode or a plate-type skin electrode. Potentials are on the order of plus and minus 0.5 mV (depending on the force of contraction), and the waveform frequency is about 1000 Hz or somewhat higher. The frequency is high enough that an oscilloscope is often used instead of an oscillograph (high-speed strip chart recorder). It may be convenient to smooth the waveform by integration and to provide an audible output to aid in locating the electrode.

Electrocardiography

The electrocardiogram (ECG) is the most familiar clinical result of biopotential measurement. The electrical signal from a pacemaker in the sinoatrial (SA) node initiates the depolarization of the muscles in the atria, causing them to contract and pump blood into the ventricles. Repolarization of the atrial muscle cells follows. The electrical signal then passes into the atrioventricular (AV) node, initiating depolarization and contraction of the ventricles and pumping blood into the pulmonary and systemic circulation. The ventricle muscle cells then repolarize. The sequence is repeated at a rate of about 72 times per minute (in a resting adult). The impulses act as a source of voltage, which generates a current flow in the torso and corresponding potentials on the skin. The potential distribution is similar to what would be observed if the heart were replaced by an electric dipole, as seen in Fig. 3.14. The dipole is located toward the left side and tilted, as is the heart. In electrocardiography, the skin potentials resulting from the torso current are sensed by electrodes at various positions on the skin. Electrodes are generally

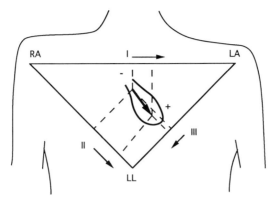

FIG. 3.14 Einthoven triangle, electric dipole vector, and ECG electrodes and leads.

located on the left arm (LA), right arm (RA), and left leg (LL). The RA-LA-LL points in the Fig. 3.14 define the Einthoven triangle. Special positions, e.g., in an arc along the chest, may be used in other examinations. The difference in potential between two electrodes corresponds to the projection of the dipole on the corresponding leg of the Einthoven triangle. The RA to LL potential difference is measured by the standard lead I, the RA to LA difference by lead II, and the LA to LL difference by lead III. Additional signals are recorded from various combinations of leads, using resistance coupling (augmented leads). The augmented voltage right arm (aVR) is $V_I - V_{III}/2$. The augmented voltage left arm (aVL) is $V_I - V_{II}/2$. The augmented voltage foot (aVF) is $V_{II} - V_I/2$. The chest (C) lead includes contributions from all three standard potentials through a resistance network. The leads are connected to the ECG machine through a switch and feed a differential amplifier and an oscillograph. The typical input impedance of the differential amplifier is 5 MΩ, and the frequency response is 0.14 to 25 Hz. The standard speed of the oscillograph is 25 mm/s and the high speed is 100 mm/s.

Figure 3.15 shows the appearance of a standard lead II waveform in a normal subject. The principal features are identified by letters. P represents

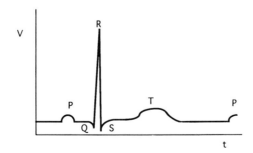

FIG. 3.15 Normal ECG waveform for lead II.

the atrial depolarization and contraction, the QRS complex corresponds to ventricular depolarization, ventricular contraction occurs between S and T, and T represents the ventricular repolarization. The amplitude of the R peak is about a millivolt. The PR interval is about 0.15 s and the $QRST$ complex extends over about 0.43 s; thus, relatively slow oscillograph recording is adequate.

Electrical interference is minimized by the differential amplifier, twisted leads, and a common mode (CM) reduction circuit. The CM circuit is a buffered balanced amplifier (two differential amplifiers with feedback) in the "neutral" path (connected to the leg).

Electroencephalography

For an electroencephalogram (EEG), many brain cortex neurons at once are recorded with electrodes fastened to the scalp. The standard 10–20 system for electrode positions is shown in Fig. 3.16. The reference electrode is usually attached to the ear. Eight to 16 channels (electrodes) are recorded simultaneously. The amplitude is only about 50 μV; therefore, careful shielding and a large CM rejection ratio (CMRR = 80 dB) in each differential amplifier are necessary to minimize interference. A 60 Hz notch filter may be used to further reduce the interference from the power line frequency, although the brain wave frequencies are below 30 Hz. The brain wave source has a high impedance and low amplitude. The differential amplifier should have an input impedance exceeding 10 MΩ and a gain of about 10^6. The amplifiers are followed by filters, e.g., high pass, low pass, and band pass, for the frequency bands of interest: delta (0.5 to 3.5 Hz), theta (4 to 7 Hz), alpha (8 to 13 Hz), and beta (over 13 Hz). A more complex analysis may be made on the waveform recorded, as in Fig. 3.16.

3.5 CHEMICAL SENSORS

The usual sensors for ions and dissolved gases are electrochemical cells that generate a potential difference between an indicator electrode and a reference electrode. The potential difference is a function of the activity of the ion (concentration modified by ion interactions) or the partial pressure (tension) of the gas and the temperature. The theory is discussed in references on electrochemistry and biomedical sensors (see, for example, Cobbold, as listed in the Bibliography at the end of this chapter). Ions of particular interest in physiology are hydrogen (as measured by pH), Na^+, K^+, and Ca^{++}. The blood gases of interest are oxygen and carbon dioxide. Blood glucose is important for patients suffering from diabetes mellitus, who may be fitted with an "artificial pancreas" to deliver insulin as needed.

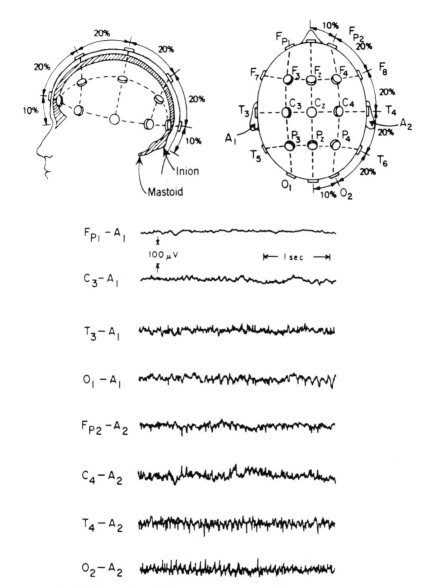

FIG. 3.16 EEG electrode positions and waveforms. (Courtesy of Medical Physics Publishing Co., Madison, Wis.)

pH

The solvent of most importance in the body is water, which is polar and weakly ionized by

$$H_2O + H_2O <-> H_3^+O + OH^-, \tag{3.17}$$

where H_3^+O is the hydrated proton or hydronium ion and OH^- is the hydroxyl ion. The equilibrium constant

$$K = \frac{(a_{H^+})(a_{OH^-})}{(a_{H_2O})^2},$$ (3.18a)

and for pure water at 25°C,

$$K_W = 1.008 \times 10^{-14},$$

hence

$$a_{H^+} = 1 \times 10^{-7}.$$ (3.18b)

The pH is defined as follows:

$$pH = -\log(a_{H^+}),$$ (3.19)

and for water is 7.0. If acid is added, the hydrogen ion activity is increased and the hydroxyl ion activity decreased, so that the activity product remains constant. Thus for acids, $pH < 7.0$, whereas for alkaline or basic solutions, $pH > 7.0$.

The emf generated in electrochemical half-cells, consisting of a metal electrode immersed in an aqueous solution containing the metal ion, is measured with respect to a reference hydrogen electrode whose potential is defined as zero at all temperatures. The standard hydrogen electrode is made of a platinum plate with an electrodeposit of the finely divided platinum-black, immersed in acid with an activity of 1 mol/l (pH = 0), with hydrogen gas at 1 atmosphere pressure bubbled over it. However, the standard hydrogen electrode is inconvenient and cannot be used at all in some solutions; therefore, it is usually replaced by another reference electrode whose potential has been measured against the hydrogen electrode. Commonly used reference electrodes are Ag/AgCl and Hg/Hg_2Cl_2 (calomel). The silver/silver-chloride electrode consists of either pure silver or silver deposited on platinum, with a porous, thin coating of silver chloride, immersed in a solution containing chloride ions, such as 0.1M HCl or KCl. The calomel electrode consists of mercurous chloride (some 0.5 cm thick) on pure mercury and immersed in saturated KCl solution. The half-cell potential of Ag/AgCl is +0.7991 V. The half-cell potential of Hg/Hg_2Cl_2 is +0.2681 V.

The indicator electrode for pH is now usually the glass electrode, shown in Fig. 3.17. Smaller pH-sensitive electrodes are available. The thin (100 μm) silicate or specially formulated glass exchanges hydrogen ions for metal ions in the glass. A potential difference is generated between the solution to be measured and the internal buffer solution, which maintains a constant pH and is often 0.1N HCl, or buffered chloride. The reference electrode may be

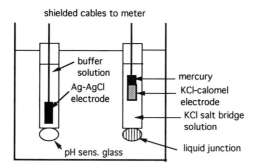

FIG. 3.17   Glass pH electrode and Hg-calomel reference.

separate or combined with the indicator electrode in one housing. In any case, the overall potential is calibrated in terms of pH by immersion in buffer solutions of known pH. A typical glass macroelectrode may have a resistance of 10^7 to 10^{10} Ω and a signal from 0 to roughly 100 mV, depending on the pH. The signal can be measured by an amplifier with an input resistance of greater than 10^{13} Ω and input leakage current of less than 10^{-13} A.

Other Ions

The concentration of the Na^+ ion can be measured with a glass electrode with a high sodium content. The concentration of the K^+ ion can be measured by a glass electrode with a high potassium content, but it is also sensitive to Na^+. The concentration of Na^+ has to be measured and a correction made to the K^+ glass electrode reading.

A liquid can be substituted for glass as an ion exchange medium. For example, K^+ concentration can be measured from the potential of an electrode where the ion exchange medium is potassium in an organic liquid. The liquid is contained in a cell with a porous disk that presents the ion exchange liquid to tissue. For measurement of Ca^{++}, the operator may use the calcium salt of didecyl phosphoric acid in dioctylphenylphosphonate. Such a cell typically has a range of 1 to 10^{-5} mol/l.

Oxygen Tension

The oxygen electrode consists of a noble metal (usually platinum) immersed in the medium to be measured and biased negatively with respect to the reference electrode. The return path may be the tissue fluid or, better, a salt bridge. A salt bridge is a glass tube containing a liquid electrolyte such as saturated KCl with membranes permeable to all ions at each end; its function is to prevent mixing of the solutions while permitting free passage of ions. A polarogram is taken by measuring the current (μA) as voltage (V) is increased. As seen in Fig. 3.18, there is an initial increase followed by a saturation region

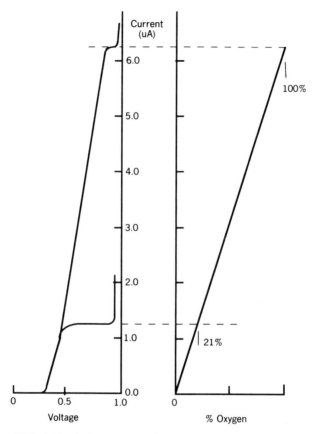

FIG. 3.18   Polarogram and calibration of oxygen sensor.

where the current is constant. The saturation current is proportional to the concentration of dissolved oxygen, so that once a suitable "plateau" is found, the voltage can be held constant while the current is calibrated against oxygen tension (pressure), often as a percentage. A problem with the bare platinum electrode is "poisoning," especially by protein in solution, resulting in a long-term drift. The more stable Clark electrode design, based on an oxygen-permeable membrane, is diagrammed in Fig. 3.19. The membrane may be Teflon 25 μm thick, and the platinum electrode may be 0.025 mm in diameter. Note that the reference electrode is inside the oxygen sensor. Microelectrodes can be fabricated that allow measurements to be made even across capillary blood vessels.

Carbon Dioxide Tension

Measurements of the partial pressure (tension) of carbon dioxide dissolved in tissue fluid or blood can also be made with a Clark-type electrode. The

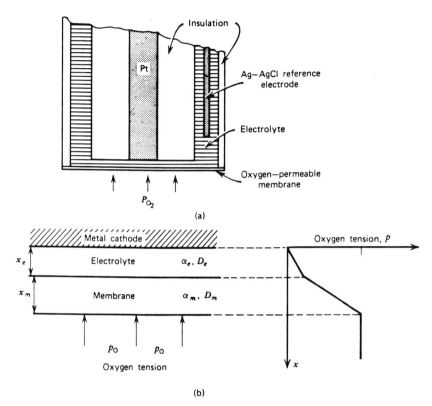

FIG. 3.19   Schematic and model of Clark oxygen electrode. (Cobbold, R. S. C. 1974. *Transducers for biomedical measurements.* New York: John Wiley & Sons.)

method is based on measuring the pH (with a glass electrode), because CO_2 dissolved in water forms the weakly dissociated carbonic acid:

$$H_2CO_3 = \alpha P_{CO_2}, \tag{3.20a}$$

where α is the solubility, and

$$H_2CO_3 <-> H^+ + HCO_3^-. \tag{3.20b}$$

A sodium bicarbonate-KCl solution is trapped in a net, and

$$pH = \frac{-\log K_1 \alpha P_{CO_2}}{a_{Na^+}}, \tag{3.21}$$

where K_1 is the dissociation constant for the reaction in equation 3.20b. Thus, the pH is proportional to the logarithm of the partial pressure of carbon dioxide.

Glucose Concentration

Figure 3.20 shows an electrode designed to measure the concentration of glucose in blood, using an immobilized enzyme (glucose oxidase). The reaction is

$$\text{Glucose} + O_2 \underset{\text{glucose oxidase}}{<->} \text{gluconic acid} + H_2O_2. \qquad (3.22)$$

An enzyme is a catalyst. The glucose concentration is proportional to the reduction in oxygen tension if the glucose concentration is not too large and the oxygen concentration in solution is large enough not to be rate limiting. Oxygen is measured by the oxygen electrode with its selective membrane. To avoid a dependence on the oxygen tension, a second electrode is incorporated, but with the enzyme inactivated by heating. The difference between the two cathode currents is used to determine the glucose concentrations.

Fiberoptic Sensors

Fiberoptic sensors, or optrodes, are being developed for measurements in vivo. They are of two kinds: direct, or plain, and indicator mediated. The plain optrode is used to measure the reflectance (or absorbance) of colored tissue compounds, or their native fluorescence, at selected wavelengths. In the indicator-mediated optrode, changes in reflectance (or absorbance) or fluorescence of a bound reagent are detected as the reagent reacts with the tissue or body fluid. A typical fiberoptic sensor has one fiber from the light source to the tissue site, and another fiber from the tissue site to filters and a detector. Only one fiber is needed for fluorescence measurements if the longer-wavelength fluorescence light is separated from the excitation light,

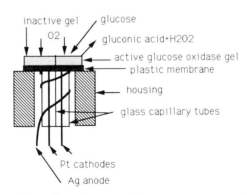

FIG. 3.20   Glucose electrode. Glucose oxidase enzyme reacts with glucose and oxygen, reducing oxygen concentration, measured with oxygen electrode. Enzyme inactivated by heat in second gel, compensates for oxygen concentration changes from other causes.

e.g., by a dichroic beam splitter. This is a partially reflecting, partially transmitting mirror with a transition from reflection to transmission at a selected wavelength.

As an example of the use of a plain optrode, consider the absorption spectra of reduced or deoxyhemoglobin and oxyhemoglobin in Fig. 3.21a, and the fiberoptic sensor shown in Fig. 3.22a. The oxygen saturation (OS) is the ratio of the amount of oxygen carried by hemoglobin in the erythrocytes in blood, to the maximum amount. The reflected light signal at 660 nm is measured and ratioed to the signal at the isobestic point of reduced and oxidized hemoglobin at 805 nm. The signal at the isobestic point occurs mostly from scattering. The ratio is insensitive to variations in refractive index, hematocrit, and other influences. A device for measuring OS is called an oximeter.

Figure 3.21b shows the excitation and emission spectra, and Fig. 3.22b is a drawing of a fiberoptic fluorescence sensor for in vivo measurements of the

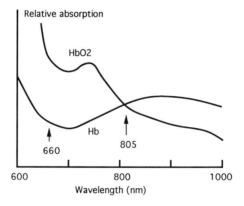

(a) Relative absorption vs wavelength for oxygenated and reduced hemoglobin.

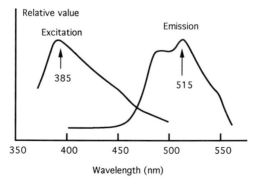

(b) Fluorescence excitation and emission spectra of oxygen-sensitive dye.

FIG. 3.21   Absorption and fluorescence properties for oxygen sensor.

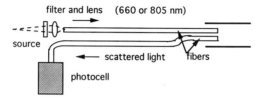

(a) Fiberoptic sensor for oxygen saturation by ratio of scattered light at 660 nm and 805 nm

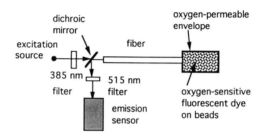

(b) Fluorescence quenching by oxygen, single fiber

FIG. 3.22   Fiberoptic sensors depending on scattered light **(a)**, and on fluorescence **(b)**.

partial pressure of oxygen, pO_2. The detection is based on the quenching by oxygen of the fluorescence of perylene dibutyrate absorbed on polystyrene beads. The beads are contained in a thin (25 μm) polypropylene tube. Excitation is at 385 nm, and emission is detected at 515 nm. Then

$$pO_2 = (\text{gain}) \, (I_o/I - 1)^m, \tag{3.23}$$

where I_o is the intensity from the scattered excitation light (or fluorescence at a wavelength outside perylene dibutyrate fluorescence). I is the intensity from the fluorescence, and m corrects for curvature in the calibration curve.

3.6   SIGNAL PROCESSING

An amplifier and the associated signal processing or conditioning circuits are chosen to match the impedance of the sensor (source) and to have a sufficient bandwidth to reproduce the waveform of the signals without introducing a lot of noise. The amplifier must also have sufficient gain, with good linearity and gain stability, to amplify the small signal from the sensor to a level sufficient to operate the display or readout device (generally 1 to 10 V).

Negative feedback is often applied to increase linearity and bandwidth, at the expense of gain.

Fourier Analysis

Signal waveforms and the transient response of sensors may be analyzed in either the frequency domain or, equivalently, in the time domain. Any periodic signal of period T can be analyzed into sums of sines and cosines in integer multiples (harmonics) of the fundamental frequency (Fourier analysis):

$$f(t) = \frac{a_0}{2} + \sum_{n=1}^{\infty} a_n \cos \omega t + b_n \sin \omega t, \tag{3.24}$$

where $a_0/2$ is the average or DC value and

$$a_n = \frac{2}{T} \int_0^T f(t) \cos n\omega t \, dt, \tag{3.25a}$$

$$b_n = \frac{2}{T} \int_0^T f(t) \sin n\omega t \, dt, \tag{3.25b}$$

or in terms of the phase

$$f(t) = \frac{a_0}{2} + \sum_{n=1}^{\infty} c_n \sin(n\omega t - f_n), \tag{3.26a}$$

where

$$c_n = \sqrt{a_n^2 + b_n^2}, \tag{3.26b}$$

$$f_n = \tan^{-1} \frac{a_n}{b_n}. \tag{3.26c}$$

The waveform obtained by adding the first four Fourier components (including the fundamental), is shown in Fig. 3.23. The fundamental frequency should be $\frac{1}{72}$ per minute, or $\frac{60}{72} = 0.8$ cycles per second (for blood pressure). However, to give the approximation with $n = 4$, the transducer and amplifier have to respond with constant gain and zero phase shift to frequencies up to at least 3.2 Hz. For more abruptly changing waveforms, many more harmonics must be used for an accurate representation. For example, an ECG may require 30 to 60 harmonics to represent adequately the *QRS* complex. Fourier analysis can be applied even to nonperiodic waveforms, but then, instead of discrete frequency *lines*, a broadened spectrum of frequencies is seen. The Fourier transform, or spectral distribution, of a single spike of negligible width is a uniform distribution across the entire range in frequencies from zero to in-

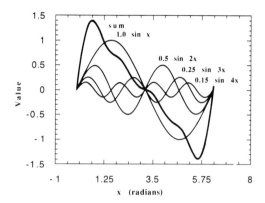

FIG. 3.23 Fourier analysis. Sum of fundamental and three harmonics as approximation of pressure pulse.

finity, but the representation may be adequate even for a limited range of frequencies. Fourier analysis shows that the entire measurement system must respond with constant gain and zero phase shift to that range of frequencies that gives adequate fidelity in the reproduction of the signal waveform for the purpose at hand.

System Response

Systems are classified according to the number of energy storage elements in the equivalent circuit. A zero order system has no energy storage element such as a capacitance or an inductance in electrical systems, or a spring or a flywheel in mechanical systems. An example is the resistive potentiometer for displacement sensing. There is no variation of gain or phase with frequency.

Many physiological measurement systems can be analyzed as first-order systems containing one energy storage element. Figure 3.24 shows the frequency responses of resistance-capacitance (RC) circuits connected as high-pass and low-pass filters. The responses of these systems are

$$A_{high} = \frac{1}{1 - j(\omega RC)^{-1}}, \tag{3.27a}$$

$$A_{low} = \frac{1}{1 + j\omega RC}. \tag{3.27b}$$

The half-power ($0.707 \times$ voltage) frequencies are f_1 (high pass) and f_2 (low pass). A bandpass filter is obtained from a low-pass filter followed by a high-pass filter ($f_1 < f_2$). A notch or stopband filter is obtained by a combination of a low-pass filter followed by a high-pass filter with $f_1 > f_2$. Faster increase

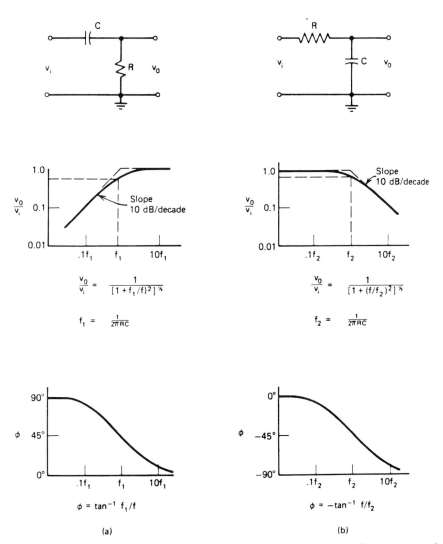

FIG. 3.24 Gain and phase response vs. frequency for first order RC high-pass and low-pass circuits.

or decrease of gain with frequency can be achieved with two or more circuits in series. The RC circuits are isolated by a buffer amplifier (an amplifier with gain of unity).

The high-pass circuit attenuates DC and low frequencies, but not high frequencies. Thus the output of a high-pass circuit reproduces the risetime of a step waveform, but not the DC component after the step. At long times, as compared with the time constant RC, it performs as a differentiator. The output from the low-pass circuit reproduces the constant level of the step, but not the risetime, and it introduces a delay. (The risetime is defined as the time for the signal to increase from 10 to 90 percent of final amplitude.) At long times the low-pass circuit acts like an integrator.

Other measurement apparatus and physiological processes can be analyzed as second-order systems, which have two energy storage elements and usually have a dissipative element for damping.

Noise and Noise Filtering

Detectors and amplifiers have several sources of noise. Johnson noise is the random variation in the current or voltage of a resistor because of random thermal motion of electrons in the resistor. The current from the resistor is given by

$$i_{n^2} = 4kTB/R, \tag{3.28}$$

where k is the Boltzmann constant, T is the absolute temperature, $B = \Delta f$ is the noise bandwidth, and R is the resistance. Note that the noise voltage does not depend on frequency; therefore, Johnson noise is "white" noise. It can be reduced by cooling the resistor.

Shot noise arises from the fundamental statistical nature of photons. It is seen, for example, in the dark current from a photomultiplier tube or image intensifier. It follows the Poisson distribution, is independent of frequency, and is important only when very low fluxes of light are involved in the measurement. The current from shot noise is given by

$$i_{n^2} = 2qiB, \tag{3.29}$$

where q is the electron charge, and i is the mean current.

Another type of noise, whose origin is not understood completely, is "1/f" noise. As indicated by the name, the amplitude of this noise decreases with increasing frequency (f). Other noise sources include the amplification process itself, and thermally induced noise may emanate from a thermal type optical detector.

A measure of noise is the noise equivalent power (NEP), the input power (e.g., optical flux) that gives a signal-to-noise ratio of unity for a specified electrical bandwidth, Δf, usually taken as 1 Hz (corresponding to an integration time of 1s). When the modulation frequency is f, the NEP is then

$$P_N(f, \Delta f) = {}^V N/|R(f)|, \tag{3.30}$$

where ${}^V N$ is the root-mean-square noise voltage, and R is the responsivity (signal voltage output per unit power input). It is obviously desirable to minimize NEP. On the other hand, one can define the normalized detectivity, a figure of merit, which increases as the signal-to-noise ratio increases. When

NEP is proportional to the square root of Δf and to the square root of the detector area (A), as is often the situation, the normalized detectivity (D^*) is expressed as

$$D^* = \frac{(A \; \Delta f)^{0.5}}{P_N} \tag{3.31}$$

Many detectors and amplifiers have a noise spectral density such as shown in Fig. 3.25. It is desirable to limit the low frequency response, and perhaps the high frequency response, or to shift the detected frequency to the midrange with a synchronized chopper and lock-in amplifier, to improve the signal-to-noise ratio.

Figure 3.26 illustrates a chopper (light source modulator) and lock-in amplifier often used for low light level optical measurements. The light source beam is modulated by a rotating chopper wheel or other device, giving a beam modulated at frequency f_s. A reference signal for frequency and phase is also generated at frequency f_r. The light source beam, after interaction in an experiment, is detected and amplified by a shielded, differential amplifier. The phase-lock loop in the reference channel extracts the phase from any waveform, and the phase can be adjusted by a control. Both experimental signal and reference are fed to a phase-sensitive detector, a multiplier that outputs a signal:

$$V = C \cos (\omega_r t + \phi) \cos(\omega_s t)$$
$$= C\{0.5 \cos[(\omega_r + \omega_s) + \phi] + 0.5 \cos [(\omega_r - \omega_s) + \phi]\}, \tag{3.32}$$

where C is an amplitude, the angular frequency is $\omega = 2\pi f$, and the phase is ϕ. The term involving the sum of frequencies is removed by the low-pass filter. The notch filters remove any contribution from pickup at the power line frequency (60 or 50 Hz), and at twice the power line frequency (120 or 100 Hz).

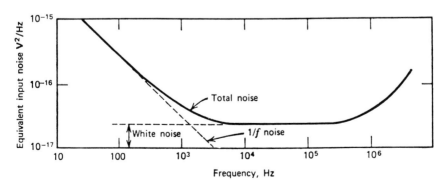

FIG. 3.25 Noise spectral density vs. frequency for a typical sensor. (Cobbold, R. S. C. 1974. *Transducers for biomedical measurements.* New York: John Wiley & Sons.)

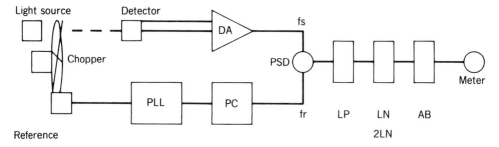

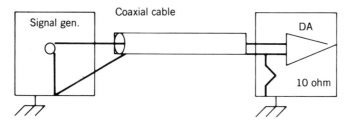

FIG. 3.26 Chopper and lock-in amplifier for noise reduction.

Other pickup is reduced by shielding the components and coupling the detector (and preamplifier if one is used) to the amplifier with shielded coaxial cable. The auto-bandpass filter further reduces bandwidth by automatically tracking on the output frequency and filtering to a reasonably narrow bandwidth around this frequency. The lock-in amplifier is basically a narrow-bandpass filter and amplifier with a frequency shifted from the predominant noise frequencies.

Although it is usually advantageous to use a transducer and an amplifier with a wide frequency bandwidth, there are situations in which a narrower bandwidth is advantageous. For example, interference from the power line or microphonics (electrical noise from vibrations) can be reduced by using a high-pass filter.

Digital Sampling

An analog or continuously varying wave can be digitized by sampling the value of the waveform at small enough time intervals (regularly spaced) to

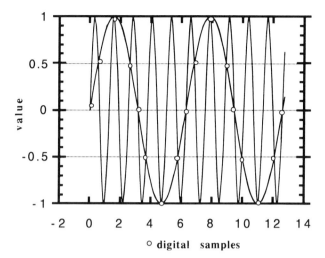

FIG. 3.27 Aliasing. The digital sampling rate chosen gives a poor representation of the high-frequency sinewave. Instead, it represents a low-frequency sinewave.

give an adequate representation of the actual variation in signal over time. The minimum sampling frequency should be 2f, where f is the highest Fourier component of interest; that is, there should be at least two samples per cycle of the highest significant frequency. Inadequate sampling frequency will give an error called *aliasing*, as illustrated in Fig. 3.27. The first waveform is sampled eight times per cycle, whereas the second is sampled roughly once per cycle. The waveform reconstructed from the sampled data is the same for both examples; it is an excellent approximation of the first (low frequency) waveform but a very poor approximation of the second (high frequency) waveform.

Impedance Considerations

Other criteria for accurate measurements (in addition to proper frequency response and linearity) is that the sensor should not perturb unduly the physiological system, and that the signal processor should not load the sensor too much. These considerations may be treated in terms of impedance. For example, the electrodes and conducting tissue in a measurement of biopotential V_1 can be treated as a source impedance (Z_s) in series with the potential generator. The input impedance of the amplifier is Z_{in}. Then the ratio of the measured voltage V_2 to the undisturbed voltage is

$$\frac{V_2}{V_1} = \frac{1}{(Z_s/Z_{in}) + 1}.$$ (3.33)

Thus the input impedance of the amplifier has to be much greater than the source impedance for all frequencies of importance.

3.7   ELECTRONIC CIRCUITS

A number of electronic circuits are used in biomedical instrumentation. It would take an entire book to discuss them in detail. Two circuits, however, the differential amplifier and the microprocessor, are discussed here.

Differential Amplifier

The differential amplifier is used in measurements of biopotentials, including the ECG and the EEG, and in any application where rejection of a common potential is necessary (e.g., to reduce interference from the capacitively coupled field around a power line). A diagram of a differential amplifier is shown in Fig. 3.28.

The output voltage signal $V_{out} = A_d(V_2 - V_1)$, where A_d is the differential voltage gain. The gain can be calculated from

$$V_1 = I_{B1}r_b + (\beta + 1)(I_{B1} + I_{B2})R_e, \tag{3.34a}$$

$$V_2 = I_{B2}r_b + (\beta + 1)(I_{B1} + I_{B2})R_e, \tag{3.34b}$$

$$V_{out} = -I_{B1}\beta R_L = -\frac{\beta R_L}{2R_b}(V_1 - V_2), \tag{3.34c}$$

$$A_d = \frac{+\beta r_L}{2r_b}, \tag{3.34d}$$

where I represents currents in the equivalent circuit and β is the current gain.

If the positive terminal of the differential amplifier is grounded, this is an ordinary inverting amplifier. If the negative terminal is grounded, it is a noninverting amplifier.

No amplifier is perfect, and there will be some common mode response. The common mode rejection ratio (CMRR) is the ratio of V_{out} when V_2 is grounded, to V_{out} when $V_2 = V_1$. It can be measured by grounding V_2 and applying a voltage V_1 to the negative terminal and measuring V_{out}. Next, V_2 is ungrounded, the input leads are shorted, the same value of V_1 is applied, and V_{out} is measured. Then CMRR is calculated from the two magnitudes of the two V_{out}s. A typical CMRR is 60 dB.

Microprocessor

A dedicated, special-purpose microprocessor is part of many modern biomedical instruments, for control as well as for measurement. It is really the core

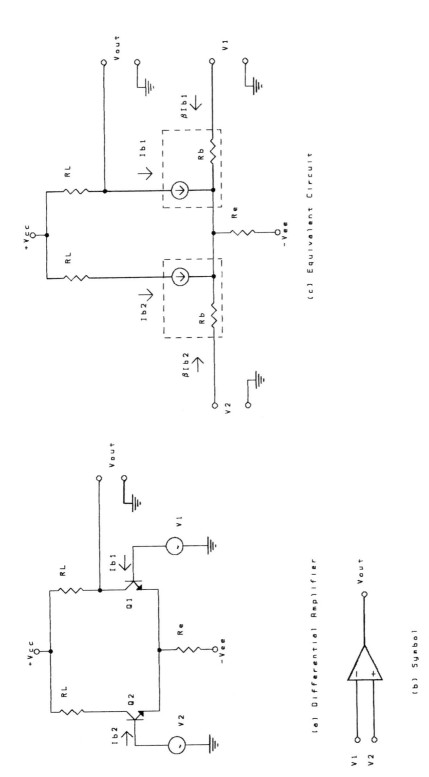

FIG. 3.28 Differential amplifier (**a**), symbol (**b**), equivalent circuit (**c**).

97

of a small digital computer. Like a computer, it may be provided with a keyboard input, as well as inputs from the sensors, a video display, and perhaps a printer or plotter.

A block diagram of a simple microprocessor is shown in Fig. 3.29. The central processing unit (CPU), memory, input unit, and output unit are integrated circuits (ICs) (chips), connected by a multiconductor data bus and a control bus. There is one conductor in each bus for every bit to be transferred. A digital oscillator provides the "clock" pulses essential to the operation of the ICs. The CPU contains an arithmetic logic unit (ALU), a timing and control module, and internal registers (accumulator, flag, program counter, and stack pointer). The memory chip consists of 8-bit registers (each bit being either 0 or 1), with a total capacity of either 1024 (1K) or 65,535 (64K) memory locations. Each separate 8-bit register is addressable, allowing transfer of data in the form of bits (0 or 1) to and from the memory. The memory may contain the program as well as space for actual data. The memory chip may be read-only memory (ROM) or random-access memory (RAM). Instructions that are not to be changed are in ROM. A special type of ROM is the programmable read-only memory (PROM), which can be programmed by a special device. An erasable, programmable ROM (EPROM) can be erased before programming, with use of a special device. The ROM retains its state when the power is off, whereas the RAM does not. Thus the instrument's program should be in ROM. RAM can be added for data.

Keyboard input may follow the ASCII code, which assigns a binary number to each decimal digit, punctuation mark, etc. A few sensing devices output digital data that can be coded as binary input. However, most biomedical sensors give an analog signal, which has to be converted to a binary number in an analog-to-digital converter (ADC). Various principles are used in ADCs; one is illustrated in Fig. 3.30. The analog voltage (V_{anal}) is applied across a voltage divider, and the voltage at each node is supplied to a threshold de-

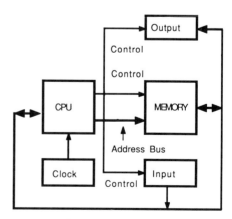

FIG. 3.29   Microprocessor block diagram.

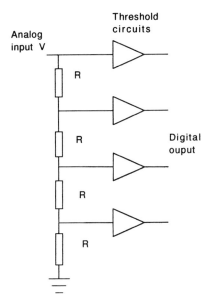

Threshold circuits

Analog input V

R

R   **Digital ouput**

R

R

FIG. 3.30   Analog-to-digital converter.

tector. If the voltage is higher than the threshold voltage, that bit is 1. If the voltage is less than the threshold voltage, that bit is 0. The ADC may analyze the input voltage into 16 to 256 channels, with each channel coded into a binary number for transmission on the bus.

The output unit may communicate with a special IC that converts binary data to data suitable for display on a video monitor or screen. It may also communicate with a printer or plotter. The output unit of the microprocessor (μP) may be used as well for control of the biomedical instrument.

BIBLIOGRAPHY

Aston, R. 1990. *Principles of biomedical instrumentation and measurement*. Columbus: Merrill Publishing Co.

Cameron, J. R., and J. G. Skofronick. 1978. *Medical physics*. New York: John Wiley & Sons.

Cobbold, R. S. C. 1974. *Transducers for biomedical measurements*. New York: John Wiley & Sons.

Cromwell, L., M. Arditti, F. J. Weibell, et. al., 1976. *Medical instrumentation for health care*. Englewood Cliffs, N.J.: Prentice-Hall.

Geddes, L. A., and L. E. Baker. 1975. *Principles of applied biomedical instrumentation*. 2d ed. New York: John Wiley & Sons.

Malmstadt, H. V., C. G. Enke, and S. R. Crouch. 1981. *Electronics and Instrumentation for Scientists*. Mass.: Benjamin/Cummings Publishing.

Rolfe, P. 1988. Review of chemical sensors for physiological measurement. *J. Biomed. Eng.* 10: 140–145.

Webster, J. G., ed. 1992. *Medical instrumentation: Application and design.* 2d ed. Boston: Houghton Mifflin.

Wilkins, E. S. 1989. Towards implantable glucose sensors: A review. *J. Biomed. Eng.* 11: 345–352.

Wolfbeis, O. S. 1991. *Fiber optic chemical sensors and biosensors.* Vol. 2. Boca Raton, Fla.: CRC Press.

CHAPTER 4

MATERIALS, PROSTHETIC AND TREATMENT DEVICES

4.0 MODELS AND PHYSIOLOGY

The biomedical engineer uses physical and mathematical models (systems of equations) to predict or control the behavior of an organ, or system of organs, and to design devices for diagnosis, therapy, or rehabilitation. To construct models, it is necessary to have a base of empirical data and, if possible, a theory of how the body system functions. Collection of data and testing of models are often performed on animals (another type of model), but sometimes human subjects are required. Animals must be treated humanely, and a human subject must give written informed consent, for both ethical and legal reasons. The study of the function, as opposed to the structure (anatomy) of organs and systems of organs or whole organisms, is the province of physiology. There are many books on physiology, and an entire course could be devoted to normal and abnormal physiology. This chapter focuses on the essentials of physiology of selected systems on which much work has been done by biomedical engineers.

4.1 BIOMATERIALS

Biomaterials are manufactured substitutes for natural tissues. They are used in implants or to convey and process body fluids such as blood. Standard design considerations may apply, such as strength and deformation, fatigue and creep, friction and wear resistance, flow resistance and pressure drop, thermal stability and expansion, electrical conductivity, optical transparency and refractive index, and so on. In addition, the material must be biocompatible and able to withstand cleaning and sterilization to minimize the risk of infection. A material is biocompatible if it evokes a minimal adverse biological response. This includes the effect of the biological environment on the material, as well as the effect of the material on the tissue. The types of materials discussed in this chapter, as well as typical applications, are summarized in Table 4.1.

Effect on Material

Materials for implanted devices should be resistant to corrosion or attack by body fluids. The following are the most suitable corrosion-resistant metals.

316L stainless steel (18% Cr–14% Ni–3% Mo, very low c, balance Fe)
Cobalt alloys (e.g., 30% Cr–7% Mo–2.5% Ni, balance Co)
Titanium and alloys

The corrosion resistance of these materials is due to an oxide surface film.

TABLE 4.1   **Types and Uses of Biomaterials**

Metals	
316L stainless steel	Bone pins, plates, joints
CoCrMo alloys	
Titanium alloys	
Ceramics	
Alumina	Bearings, valves
Carbon	
Calcium phosphate	
Polymers	
Silicones	Cartilage and tendon replacement
Polyethylene, etc.	Tubing, coatings, sutures, breast prostheses, adhesives
Polyamides (nylon)	
Acrylics	
PTFE (Teflon)	
Polyurethane	
Composites	
Ceramic/metal	Joint parts, similar to bone
Ceramic/polymer	
Ceramic coating	

Although galvanic and stress corrosions are small, metals are not completely inert. Yet metallic pins and plates, for example, have been used for years. Ceramics are resistant to corrosion in the tissue environment. They have good strength in compression and are hard, and thus wear resistant, but brittle. In most respects, ceramics are inert in the biological environment. Polymers tend to weaken with chemical action and time, and swelling and leaching may be observed (migration of liquid into the biomaterial or migration of solid or liquid components out into the tissue). High-density polyethylene is inert and resistant to deterioration, as is polypropylene. Rigid polyvinyl chloride may become brittle as plasticizers leach out. Polyesters such as polyethylene ter-epthalate are susceptible to hydrolysis and loss of tensile strength, but Dacron cloth is used for suturing heart valves into tissue. Polyamides (nylon) absorb water and irritate tissue and may lose tensile strength. Silicone rubber (e.g., Silastic, dimethyldichlorosilane rubber with silica filler and polymerized by stannous octate), which is inert and little affected by tissue and body fluids, is used in many medical devices. Polytetrafluoroethylene (PTFE) (Teflon) is inert and not affected in solid form, but small particles may cause tissue irritation. Polymethylmethacrylate (PMMA) (Plexiglass or Lucite or PMMA adhesive), an acrylic, may be deteriorated by heat sterilization (exhibiting crazing and/or loss of strength). The adhesive or cement is often used to fasten metallic joint replacements into bone, but there is appreciable heat production during curing. Sutures are of two types: absorbable and nonabsorbable. The absorbable types are catgut or chromic treated catgut (basically collagen); they have little tensile strength after a few days. The nonabsorbable type includes silk, polyamide, polyethylene terepthalate, and PTFE. Strength is well maintained, except by nylon multifilament, which has little strength after 6 months (and also causes a significant tissue reaction). Composites (e.g., cermets, ceramic plus metal) should be similar in chemical resistance to each of the components. However, a ceramic-coated metal (such as may be desirable for wear resistance or low friction) should respond like a ceramic. Composites of fibers strong in tension, with a matrix strong in compression, combine strength, toughness, and stiffness and may permit parts to be made lighter or stronger.

Effects on Tissue

It is necessary to evaluate potential responses of tissue to contact with bio-materials. These include thrombosis and hemolysis, inflammation and adaptation, infection, carcinogenesis, and hypersensitivity.

Thrombosis. Coagulation of blood is an important consideration in the use of implants and in the use of tubing and other devices that will contain blood. The product of coagulation is a clot. If the clot is inside a blood vessel it is called a thrombus, and if the clot moves it is called an embolus. Sometimes clotting is deliberately induced (e.g., in the Dacron cloth that serves for suturing in a heart valve replacement), to form a nonthrombogenic surface once emplaced. Normally, however, materials are chosen that do not easily form clots. The best surface is the intima of a blood vessel. Arterial or venous grafts may be taken from the patient's own body, but tissue rejection limits the use of natural blood vessels from another person or species (xenografts). Some biological materials, e.g., collagenous porcine heart valves, have been used after chemical treatment to suppress immune response, and these are compatible with blood. Smooth surfaces such as glass, PMMA, polyethylene, and stainless steel are good choices. In some cases, heparin may have to be added to the blood.

Hemolysis. Disruption of erythrocytes (hemolysis) may occur in response to contact with foreign materials, or through mechanical stress. Turbulent flow and shear stresses above 1500 to 3000 dyne/cm^2 can cause hemolysis. Hemolysis can also occur if the red blood cells are immersed in a hypotonic solution, e.g., distilled water. Hemolysis does not appear to be a significant problem with the biomaterials discussed, as long as the shear stresses are low.

Inflammation. Inflammation is a generalized response to tissue injury or destruction, such as occurs in surgical implantation. The classic signs of inflammation are redness (rubor), swelling (tumor), heat (calor), and pain (dolor). Vasodilation occurs because of the activation of factor XII (Hageman factor), a chemical involved in the coagulation process, probably because of contact with collagen or a foreign protein or other material. This activation results in the release of kinins, which cause vasodilation and an increase in permeability of the endothelial cells of the capillaries. An increased supply of blood enters the capillary bed, plasma escapes through the walls, platelets and erythrocytes tend to adhere, blood flow becomes sluggish, and the tissue area appears red. The increased permeability of the capillary endothelium allows fluids to escape into the extravascular space. Normally, excess fluid is drained by lymphatic vessels, but these may be constricted or blocked by cell fragments or the original trauma. Edema, and thus swelling, result. Pain may be produced from the effect of edema on deep pain receptors, or by direct action of the kinins on nerve ends. Local heating may be associated with local disturbances of fluid flow and increased cellular activity. Pyrogens (bacterial debris, tissue necrosis, and fine particles) may cause systemic fever even without infection.

Adaptation. Neutrophils migrate to the wound site within minutes to hours, and persist for days (or longer if accompanied by infection). They are transported by the blood and then penetrate the endothelium and collect in the wound. Eosinophils and macrophages, including the multinuclear giant cells, also migrate to the site. The leucocytes digest and remove dead cells and foreign material by phagocytosis. Lymphocytes may also appear, presumably as an immune response to foreign material. The leucocytes, cell debris, and fluids form an exudate (pus) that must be drained to allow wound healing. After removal of dead cells, the next stage in the healing process is "remodeling," starting with formation of granulation tissue. This newly formed tissue has a pebbly appearance. The "pebbles" are capillary and arteriole loops or buds that form in intact tissue and eventually grow into the disturbed volume and provide the microcirculation. New cells arise from mitosis of the cells present. In addition, mucopolysaccharides and collagen are synthesized, mostly by fibroblasts, forming scar tissue. The scar acts as a scaffold or matrix for the remodeling of the tissue, which takes 1 to 2 weeks in the absence of continual irritation by the implanted material. The inflammatory response ends with encapsulation of the wound by mature scar tissue, which is relatively acellular. The thickness of the capsule depends on the degree of initial trauma and any continuing reactivity of the implant, such as production of small particles by wear or corrosion, or chemical reactivity. For example, the neointima in an implanted vascular prosthesis with an open, connected pore structure proceeds by clotting, granulation of tissue, and penetration of the pores by vascular tissue until the inner surface is covered as well.

Infection and Sterilization. It has been stated that there is a race between regenerating tissue and bacteria for sites on or near an implant. Infection of implanted biomaterial is serious and usually requires surgical removal of the implant. In addition to being clean and pyrogen free, an implant (or any material contacting a wound or blood) must be sterile. Methods of sterilization are as follows:

1. Cold solution
2. Dry heat
3. Moist heat (steam)
4. Gas
5. Radiation

Cold (room temperature) solutions are commercial preparations, such as Cidex, which usually contain formaldehyde or glutaraldehyde. The part is allowed to soak 1 to 3 hours.

Dry heat consists of heating at 320°F to 350°F for 0.5 to 2 hours (time and temperature vary inversely). Moist heat is applied in an autoclave; temperature is 250°F to 270°F for 2 to 15 minutes, varying inversely (higher temperature for a shorter time). Gas sterilization is usually performed with ethylene oxide, 400 to 1200 mg/l, 1 to 24 hours, from room temperature to 130°F. Radiation may be via energetic electrons or gamma rays, e.g., 2 to 4 Mrad, at room temperature. Irradiation is performed by the manufacturer, and the material is sealed in a container until ready for use. The choice of sterilizing method depends on its effect on the biomaterial, as well as time required or convenience. A test culture is usually taken periodically to be sure the solution or procedure is still effective.

Carcinogenesis. Cancer may be induced by exposure to chemical carcinogens or foreign bodies (FB), or by mechanical irritation. There is evidence from animal studies that pure nickel and nickel compounds, cobalt metal, and certain compounds of chromium, iron, titanium, and manganese are carcinogenic (but the pure metals are not). Other metallic carcinogens are cadmium, lead, and beryllium. However, alloys such as used in implants, and even pure titanium, do not seem to be carcinogenic in humans. Of course, the latent period may be 20 years, and cancers so induced may not yet have been diagnosed. Ceramics, perhaps because of their low solubilities, do not seem to be carcinogenic. Polymers too are usually inert, but leaching of fillers or plasticizers should be considered for carcinogenic potential. Vinyl chloride is a significant procarcinogen, as are polycyclic aromatic hydrocarbons and halogenated hydrocarbons. FB or solid-state carcinogenesis has been observed in animals with implants, even when the implant is inert chemically. The induction risk increases with size of the implant, and, strangely enough, a less inflammatory response is coupled with a greater risk of FB carcinogenesis. Porosity with pores larger than 2.2 μm reduces the risk of FB carcinogenesis. The mechanism may be an alteration of the immediate physiological environment that favors growth of malignant cells, because of altered geometry or chemical or electrical effects. Induction of cancer by implants is rare in humans, and its rate might be reduced even more by keeping the implant as small as possible.

Hypersensitivity. FBs can induce a specific hypersensitivity or allergic response from the immune system. This is a cell-mediated, delayed hypersensitivity to antigens on the surface of the FB, but may be widely disseminated in the body if fine particles are released to the lymphatics or blood.

Polymers induce little hypersensitivity unless they are made of processed natural tissue. Ceramics and composites seem to be immunologically inert. Metals may induce a response, perhaps because dissolved metal ions combine with organic molecules such as albumin to form haptens, which are immunologically active. Dermatitis is an example of a hypersensitivity reaction to contact of skin with certain metals such as nickel, chromium (as chromate), cobalt, and even gold and platinum. Another example is inflammation and necrosis resulting from implanted devices made of nickel or cobalt alloys. However, data are sparse and testing methods should be improved.

Systemic Effects. Most effects of implants are local, but dissolved metal ions and fine particles may be transported in the lymph and blood and thus have systemic effects, including potential carcinogenesis or hypersensitivity. Blood in contact with synthetic materials or subjected to hemolysis or thrombus formation in an external apparatus may also produce systemic effects. Certain elements such as iron are essential for normal body functioning, but excess ions of these elements (resulting from corrosion, for example) must be excreted or they may be toxic. Thus the systemic effects of implants, as well as extracorporeal processing, should be considered in evaluating bicompatibility.

4.2 ARTIFICIAL HIP JOINT

The mechanical properties of soft tissues are characterized by a nonlinear stress-strain relationship. These tissues are not elastic, but after repeated loading and unloading cycles, the stress-strain loop is repeatable. The loading and unloading portions are not coincident; that is, there is hysteresis. Soft tissues exhibit viscoelasticity: after sudden stretching, the stress gradually decreases with time (stress relaxation).

Bone is an inhomogeneous, anisotropic, viscoelastic material. Figure 4.1 plots stress versus strain, at different strain rates, for axial compression of cortical bone (human femur). For most purposes, however, it is sufficient to assume that bone is linearly elastic so that

$$T_{ij} = C_{ijkl} E_{k1}, \tag{4.1}$$

where T is the stress tensor, E is the infinitesimal strain tensor, and C is the fourth-order elasticity tensor. Some values for the elements of the elasticity tensor and other mechanical properties of bone are given in the *Handbook of Bioengineering* (see Skalak and Chien in the Bibliography at the end of this chapter).

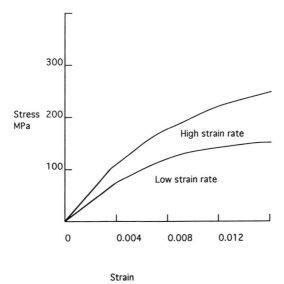

FIG. 4.1 Strain rate dependence of stress-strain curve for cortical bone.

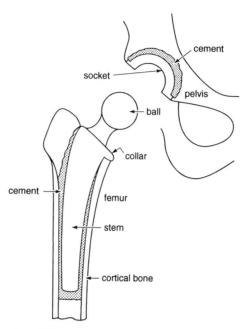

FIG. 4.2 Diagram of artificial hip joint. The socket is also known as the acetabular component.

The mechanical behavior of other tissues are also given in the *Handbook*, e.g., for articular cartilage, tendons, and ligaments.

An example of the use of biomaterials is replacement of a joint by metal and polymer. Figure 4.2 is a diagram of a total hip joint replacement. The femoral component is made of either titanium or cast cobalt-chromium alloy, cemented in the bone with PMMA adhesive. The acetabular component receives less stress, but is also made of titanium or cobalt-chromium alloy, fixed with PMMA which also fills the space between bone and metal. The bearing material is typically high-density polyethylene. The proper design of a strong, lightweight replacement and its effect on the bone may require stress analysis by a mathematical model or a polarized plastic stress test.

4.3 FEEDBACK CONTROL

Many systems in the body, and in external apparatus, depend on feedback control.

A generalized schematic diagram of a closed-loop feedback control system is given in Fig. 4.3. The output variable is T_o (e.g., actual temperature) and the reference variable is T_r (e.g., desired temperature). The output-input transfer function or "gain" of the effector or controlled system (e.g., a heater

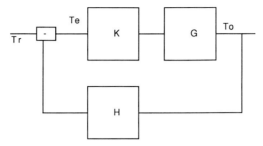

FIG. 4.3 Feedback control scheme. T_o is the existing value of the quantity to be controlled, and T_r is the desired value. The error signal is T_e. G is the transfer function or gain of the effector, H, the gain of the sensor, and K, the gain of the controller.

and water bath) is G. The controller gain is K. A sensor (e.g., of temperature), with transfer function or gain H, is located in a feedback loop. The controller may respond to the instantaneous error or difference signal T_e, or more complicated control schemes may be involved, such as multiple inputs or the history and predicted future course. In any event, the controller has to allow for time delays in signal propagation time and response time of the effector. If a rapidly varying control is desired, the frequency responses of G, H, and K have to be considered.

Negative feedback is usually applied, as positive feedback leads in to an ever-increasing output. The output variable, T_o, is related to the error signal, T_e, by

$$\delta T_o = KG\, \delta T_e \tag{4.2}$$

and the error signal

$$T_e = T_r - HT_o; \tag{4.3}$$

hence

$$\delta T_o = \frac{KG}{1 + KGH}\, T_r. \tag{4.4}$$

In developing a feedback control system, one must consider accuracy and stability. The system tries to minimize error between the desired value of a variable, such as temperature, and the value actually existing. Accuracy of following changes in the desired or reference value is improved by increasing the overall gain, but this often leads to instability, in which the variable oscillates around the desired value. Not only must the system be stable, but it must also have an adequate margin of stability—a problem when there are significant delays, as in the neuromuscular system. The stability is improved at low gain, and a compromise must be made. Linear systems can be analyzed for stability in terms of the Nyquist criterion.

Assume the heater-water bath in the example has a transfer function (G) of 1°C per watt input. Power must be supplied to increase the temperature and to make up for heat losses. Also assume the thermocouple temperature gauge transfer function is $H = 50~\mu V$ per °C.

To control at $T_o = 50$°C above ambient, the sensor voltage should be 2.5 mV, and T_r should be 2.5 mV (if there is no amplification in H). Then the transfer function (K) of the controller should be 20 W/mV. The heater power is large while T_e is large, and tapers off to zero when $T_e = 0$.

4.4 NEUROMUSCULAR CONTROL

Muscle contraction, and therefore movement of the bones connected to the muscle, is controlled naturally by feedback involving sensors and the central nervous system (CNS). Control of skeletal muscle by external electrical stimulation is currently used to rehabilitate paraplegic and quadraplegic patients.

Effector

Muscle is the effector in the biomedical engineering problem considered here. Muscles, especially those involved in moving limbs, occur in opposing pairs (agonist and antagonist) and must be coordinated to achieve a desired motion. Other muscles may also be involved, e.g., to stabilize a joint.

As discussed in Chapter 2, skeletal muscle fibers are multinucleated cells running the length of a muscle, from origin to insertion. The fibers are bundled into groups connected by a membrane, and groups are bundled to give the full cross section of that muscle. Contraction, hence shortening of the fiber, is accomplished in the sarcomeres. Muscle contraction is rather efficient: about 70 percent of the energy in adenosine triphosphate (ATP) can be converted into mechanical work. The reduction of glucose to form ATP is about 50 percent efficient. The synthesis of ATP from fat, carbohydrates, and protein occurs through oxidative phosphorylation in the mitochondria (requiring oxygen), or breakdown of glucose to pyruvic and lactic acids (glycosis). The muscle will fatigue if ATP is consumed more rapidly than it can be replenished. Contraction can also occur by the anerobic breakdown of glucose to lactic acid. The glucose is obtained either from the blood or from the breakdown of glycogen in the muscle. However, the muscle fatigues more rapidly in such a case than in aerobic synthesis of ATP. A period of rest must be allowed for recovery from fatigue.

The relationship between muscle length and the force (tension, pull) exerted can be more readily studied in the sarcomere. Figure 4.4 shows the tension versus length of the sarcomere, as well as the tension of the whole muscle versus length, as compared with the resting length l_o. The tetanized

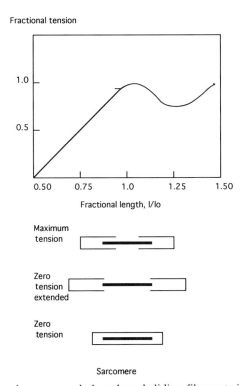

FIG. 4.4   Tension vs. muscle length and sliding filaments in sarcomere.

curve was measured for muscle in isometric (constant length) contraction. Maximum tension is exerted at the resting length. The muscle is overextended at greater lengths and the force is reduced. Likewise, as the sarcomere fibrils slide over each other, the available tension decreases until finally no force can be exerted.

Normally, contraction is initiated by the impulse from a motor neuron, called an *alpha neuron*. One neuron may stimulate many muscle cells. The neuron and associated muscle fibers is called a *motor unit*. Muscles used for coarse tasks are composed of relatively few motor units, and each motor unit has many, perhaps hundreds, of fibers per neuron. In fine-control muscles there are many motor units, each with relatively few muscle fibers (approximately 10). More force is generated by activating or "recruiting" more motor units. The force is also altered by the frequency of the nerve impulses, as illustrated in Fig. 4.5. For low frequencies, the motor unit fibers "twitch," that is, contract and then relax. If the frequency of impulses is increased, the muscle cannot relax completely between them, and the contractive force tends to build up, but with oscillations at the frequency of stimulation—a condition termed *unfused tetanus*. At still higher frequencies, the smooth curve labeled

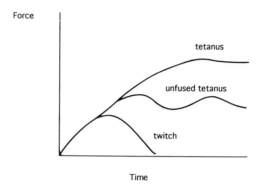

FIG. 4.5 Muscle contraction vs. frequency of stimulation. Single pulse, one twitch. Higher frequency, unfused tetanus. High frequency, tetanus (continuous contraction).

tetanus is observed, and the force is roughly twice that exerted at the maximum of a single twitch.

There is a time delay in the conduction of the nerve impulse from the CNS (spinal cord) to the muscle of 10 ms or so, depending on the specific nerve and the distance of travel. There is a delay at the neuromuscular junction as the neurotransmitter substance is released and diffuses to the other side. Delays also occur corresponding to conduction of the nerve impulse within the muscle, the release and diffusion of calcium ions, and the splitting of ATP. Contraction is a chemical process, so contractive force does not develop instantaneously but increases over some tens of milliseconds. There is a latency period after stimulation with an external electrical voltage, and even a small relaxation before the force builds.

The situation is further complicated by the existence of two types of muscle fibers: fast-twitch and slow-twitch, as shown in Fig. 4.6. Fast-twitch fibers have a type of myosin that is good for rapid splitting of ATP and contraction of the muscle, with a short latency period and associated with high strength and rapid response, but for a limited time. Slow-twitch fibers have a long latency period, because of a slow neuromuscular conduction system, and are associated with endurance activities such as standing. Most muscles have a

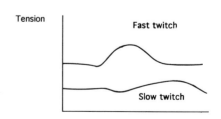

FIG. 4.6 Fast and slow twitch muscle fibers. Tension vs. time after stimulation.

mix of fast-twitch and slow-twitch fibers, and their activities can be enhanced by appropriate training or exercise (weight lifting for fast-twitch, endurance activities for slow-twitch). The metabolically dependent contraction process is also affected by physiological and environmental factors such as temperature. Speed of contraction, muscle strength, and endurance are decreased as the temperature of the muscle is decreased below normal (37°C, approximately). Another consideration is fatigue: repeated contractions lead to a decrease in the speed of contraction.

A mathematical model must be constructed for the muscle before a control scheme can be designed. The model may be based purely on empirical data, or there may be a theoretical relationship. The Hill relationship between tension (T) and velocity (v) is empirical:

$$(T + a)(v + b) = (T_o + a)b, \qquad (4.5)$$

where a and b are constants fitted to data and T_o is the maximum tension, or

$$\frac{v}{v_o} = \frac{1 - T/T_o}{1 + T/kT_o}, \qquad (4.6)$$

where $v_o = bT_o/a$ is the shortening velocity under no load, and $k = aT_o = b/v_o$. For most muscles, $0.15 < k < 0.25$. Figure 4.7 illustrates the inverse hyperbolic relationship between muscle shortening velocity (v) and constant-

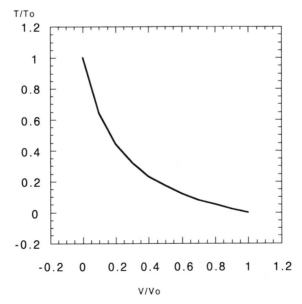

FIG. 4.7   Hill tension-velocity relationship. *To* is maximum tension. *Vo* is maximum velocity.

force or isotonic load (T), calculated with parameters a and b fitted to data for a particular muscle. More complicated models take into account not only the load but also the recruitment magnitude, fraction of slow-twitch fibers, initial length, and temperature, and attempt to derive the constants.

Sensors

The body's natural sensors include the pacinian capsule, the muscle spindle, and the Golgi tendon organ. The pacinian sensor is a capsule with a free nerve ending inside; it responds to pressure, generating a stream of nerve impulses. Like many other biological sense organs, it exhibits accommodation: after being exposed to a certain pressure for a period of time, it stops sending nerve impulses until the pressure is changed. The muscle spindle, a fibrous structure with a nerve, measures changes in muscle length. The CNS recalibrates the baseline for the muscle length change. The Golgi tendon organ transmits information about force to the CNS.

Artificial sensors may be used in prosthetics to measure displacement or position, velocity, and force or pressure. Among those used for neuromuscular control are the potentiometer, the Hall-effect transducer, the variable displacement differential transformer, the digital shaft encoder (optical), the elastic resistor (a cord that can be stretched and that changes its resistance when its length changes), the capacitive transducer, and the resistive strain gauge.

Controller

The natural controller is the cell body of the alpha motor neuron, which receives (through synapses) and integrates impulses from many other neurons in the CNS. The synapses may be excitatory or inhibitory. A single nerve impulse is usually insufficient to cause the motor neuron to develop its own action potential. Instead, there must be many impulses in a short time, or many impulses from other neurons. In addition, the synapses closer to the axon hillock have a greater effect than those more distant. The weighted summation of all excitatory and inhibitory impulses determines whether the alpha motor neuron conducts. The actual working of the natural muscle controller is very complex, taking into account voluntary decisions, feedback from sensors, coordination between different muscles, and so forth.

Artificial control is based on electrical stimulation of the alpha motor neuron. The stimulation or "shock" may be applied to the nerve or intramuscularly—or even to the skin, although problems with burns may occur. The control action may be to keep the muscle either entirely contracted or relaxed. For movement, however, proportional control of tension is desired. Although a muscle may be driven to fused tetanus at a sufficiently high artificial stimulation frequency (up to 300 Hz), this is not desirable. The neurotransmitter in the synapses is depleted and the muscle fatigues rapidly.

Instead, it is desirable to stimulate at a low frequency (5 to 60 Hz) and rotate the motor units stimulated and thus recruited. Natural recruitment rotation is asynchronous in nature, but sequential stimulation can be used, changing the part of the muscle contracting, to lessen fatigue, and adjusting the number of motor units recruited as necessary to develop the force required.

A digital computer or microprocessor controller designed by Petrofsky and Phillips to control a single cat muscle is shown in Figure 4.8. There are two programs, one for isometric contraction and one for isotonic contraction. In isometric contraction, where a force is exerted but no motion occurs, the system uses a combination of stimulating electrodes and DC blocking electrodes connected to the microprocessor through digital-to-analog (D-A) convertors. Sensory feedback from a strain gauge is passed through an A-D convertor. The program sets stimulation frequencies and recruitment patterns (by changing the anodal block voltage) with the slowly contracting motor units recruited first for light loads, and the faster contracting units recruited in sequence. A plot of the program is shown in Fig. 4.9, in terms of the stimulation frequencies and recruitment percentage hence the resulting tension versus time (in percentage of time to fatigue). As the time to fatigue approaches, the stimulation frequency and percentage recruitment must both be increased to maintain the tension. The time to fatigue depends on the load: at small loads (less than about 20 percent of maximum) the isometric contraction can be maintained indefinitely, whereas at heavier loads the endurance time decreases drastically.

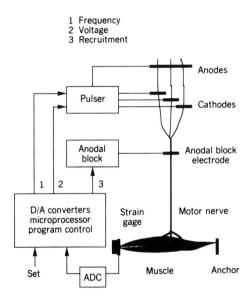

FIG. 4.8 Microprocessor control of isometric muscle contraction. (From Petrofsky, J. S., and C. A. Phillips, 1986. Closed loop control of movement of skeletal muscle. *Critical Reviews in Biomedical Engineering* 13(1): 35–95.)

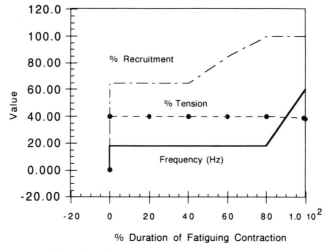

FIG. 4.9 Program for isometric contraction.

For constant velocity isotonic contraction, a different program is needed. The program is more complicated than that for isometric conduction, as one needs to know not only the load but also the velocity and the position. The delay in propagation of the impulse through the nerve and muscle (about 15 ms) and the further delay (also about 15 ms) for buildup to full tension must be taken into account. Petrofsky and Phillips took the successive approximation approach. The algorithm, diagrammed in Fig. 4.10, is based on first stimulating the muscle a moderate amount, measuring the velocity of con-

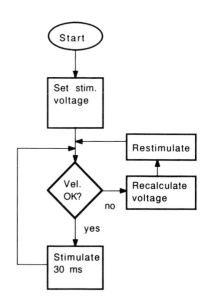

FIG. 4.10 Velocity and load program for isotonic contraction.

traction, calculating the load from the Hill (or similar) relationship, and then adjusting the level of stimulation to approach the desired velocity. For more information on the model, see the review article by these authors listed in the Bibliography at the end of this chapter.

A system was built and tested, based on the microprocessor control scheme, to enable paraplegic patients to walk and stand. At its present state of development, the device consists of an articulated leg brace fitted with sensors, level sensors on the hips, stimulating and blocking electrodes, and a small portable computer programmed for the subject to stand up or sit down, stand in one position, lift one leg and put it down, lift the other leg and put it down, etc., for coordinated walking. The programmed sequences are turned on and off by sensors in the shoulder. Many other functions had to be considered as well. The system is still under development but has already achieved some success.

4.5 HEART-LUNG MODELS AND DEVICES

Normal Heart Rhythm

The normal resting heartbeat is initiated by the "pacemaker" tissue of the sinoatrial (S-A) node at the right atrium. The electrical impulse is conducted to the atria (causing them to contract simultaneously) and to the atrioventricular (A-V) node. After a delay, the impulse passes through the bundle of His to the ventricles. The heart rate set by the natural pacemaker is 150 beats per minute, but sensors for blood pressure are inhibitory and reduce the normal rate for the body and mind at rest to about 70 beats per minute. On the other hand, exercise and the effect of noradrenalin and adrenalin in emotional excitement will increase heart rate up to some 210 beats per minute. Other effects can also influence the heart rate. Although the heart output does increase with heart rate at first, at high rates the heart chambers cannot fill with blood completely and the stroke volume and heart output tend to decrease.

Arrhythmias

Problems with generation of impulses in the S-A node (sinus arrest) or conduction of impulses (blocks of various degrees of severity), or a lack of coordination of the muscles (fibrillation) result in various heart arrhythmias. There may be no beat, or the heart rate may be too slow (brachycardia) or too fast (tachycardia). Some of these abnormalities can be treated with drugs, and/or an artificial pacemaker. The function of a pacemaker is to generate electrical pulses to stimulate contraction of the atria or ventricles (or both) at an adjustable pace (depending on physiological demand). It must not generate a pulse if the beat does occur naturally. An electrical shock from a defibrillator may stop fibrillation in an emergency.

TABLE 4.2 Pacemaker Parameters

Parameter	Specification
Rate	40–170 beats/min
Amplitude	5 V approx.
Pulse width	0.1–2 ms
Atrial sensitivity	0.75–3 mV
Ventricular sensitivity	1.0–5 mV
A, V refractory period	150–300 ms
Program modes	Usually DDD

Pacemaker. The typical artificial pacemaker is implantable, powered by a long-life lithium battery or a thermocouple heated by a plutonium-238 alpha radiois-otope source and connected by high quality leads to the heart. Modern pace-makers may be only several millimeters in diameter and weight 40 g. Typical properties are listed in Table 4.2. A pacemaker with leads is shown in Fig. 4.11.

The lead arrangements depend, among other things, on the program ca-pability of the pacemaker. It is now possible to install a pacemaker with intravenously introduced leads in a patient under local anesthesia. The leads are insulated, and each is provided with a fastener on the end. A unipolar lead embeds the cathode in the myocardium and the anode elsewhere in the body. A bipolar lead has both electrodes in the myocardium, typically spaced 15 to 30 mm apart. The pacemaker and leads are electrostatically shielded and electrically filtered to minimize interference from external sources.

The inhibited-demand pacemaker responds to spontaneous activity and resets the pulse train in synchronization with the spontaneous pulse. No pulses are generated when the natural rate is higher than the basic pacemaker rate. When the spontaneous (natural) rate is higher than the pacemaker rate, the

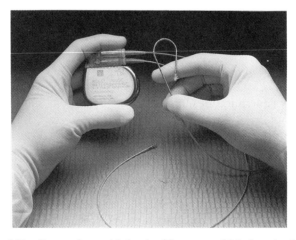

FIG. 4.11 Pacemaker, with leads. (Courtesy of Medtronic, Inc.)

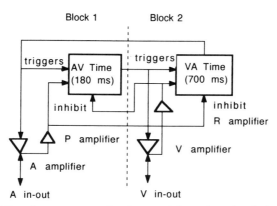

FIG. 4.12 DDD pulse generator. **Block 1:** atrial sensing circuit detects natural or stimulated atrial contraction and triggers ventricular stimulating pulse if ventricular activity is not detected within a preset time (180 ms). **Block 2:** ventricular sensing circuit detects natural or stimulated ventricular contraction and triggers an atrial pulse if no atrial activity is detected after another preset time (700 ms).

triggered-demand pacemaker will stimulate during the refractory interval of the heart muscle and no contraction will occur. The goal is to develop a pacemaker that will respond to physiological variables, as does the natural heart function, so that the heart rate can adjust automatically.

An improved design is the DDD pacemaker. A block diagram of a DDD pulse generator and sensing circuit is given in Fig. 4.12. Both atrial and ventricular pulses are detected, and both atrial and ventricular stimulation is possible. In Block 1, the atrial circuit detects both natural and stimulated atrial contraction and triggers a ventricular stimulating pulse if a ventricular pulse does not occur naturally within 180 ms. In Block 2, a ventricular-pulse–sensing circuit detects both natural and stimulated ventricular contraction and triggers an atrial-stimulating pulse if no atrial pulse is detected within 700 ms.

Defibrillator. Electrical defibrillation establishes a uniform state of ventricular excitability by sending a substantial fraction of heart muscle into the refractory state. A large electrical shock is applied to the chest. Although the action is similar to that of a pacemaker, about 20 A and pulse durations of 5 to 10 ms are required with large (7.5 cm) electrodes on the skin, with conductivity pads (much of the current bypasses the heart). Because the skin and tissue resistance varies, it is standard practice to control the energy applied (about three-fourths of the energy stored) instead of the current. The energy is stored in an R-L-C (or RC) circuit and then discharged.

Circulation

Most of the mechanical work done by the heart is spent in overcoming the frictional resistance of the arterioles and capillaries of the systemic circulation,

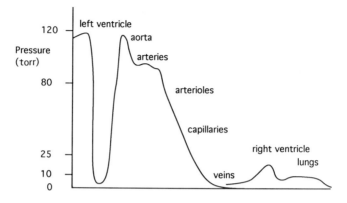

(a) Pressure (torr) in blood vessels

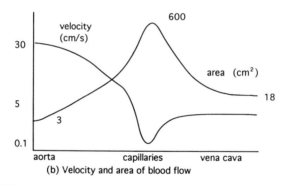

(b) Velocity and area of blood flow

FIG. 4.13   Pressure, velocity, and area of blood flow.

as seen from the pressure drops in Fig. 4.13, which also graphs the blood flow velocity, and flow cross-sectional area. Much research in biomedical engineering has been concerned with modeling blood flow dynamics, taking into account the non-Newtonian viscosity of the blood and the geometry and properties of the blood vessels, including distensibility. The viscosity of blood over the normal range of flow velocities is about 3 to 4×10^{-3} Pa s, but it increases with hematocrit and decreases with increasing temperature. The viscosity is higher at very low flow rates. For comparison, the viscosity of water is about 1×10^{-3} Pa s.

Turbulent flow can occur in the aorta for a short time near systole, and around obstructions in the bloodstream. However, blood flow is usually laminar and can be described by Poiseuille's law:

$$Q' = \Delta P \frac{1}{\eta} \frac{R^4}{L}, \tag{4.7}$$

where Q' is the flow rate, ΔP is the difference in pressure from inlet to outlet of the tube, η is the viscosity, R is the inner radius, and L is the length of the tube. Actually, Poiseuille's law applies to straight, rigid circular tubes; more exact models would take into account the elasticity of the tube walls, bends, etc.

Table 4.3 lists radii (R) of blood vessels. Although the total flow area increases as the vessels branch, the R^4 dependence overrides this and the small radius capillaries are responsible for a significant pressure drop, as the total flow rate has to be maintained. Also listed in Table 4.3 are the mean pressure (P) in the vessel and the force per unit length of tube, $T = RP$. The small radius allows even the very thin-walled and weak capillaries to withstand the blood pressure in them without rupture, whereas the large aorta has a relatively large tension per unit length and the walls are thick and reinforced with fibrous and muscular tissue.

Gas Exchange

Oxygen diffuses from blood to cell though the endothelial cell wall of the capillaries, and through the intercellular fluid, as a result of the difference in partial pressure of oxygen in blood and tissue. Because the diffusion distance is only several tens of micrometers, the body cells have to lie close to a capillary. According to Cameron and Skofronick (listed in this chapter's Bibliography), in skeletal muscle there are some 190 capillaries per square millimeter in a cut through the muscle, or a 190-mm length of capillaries in 1 mm^3 of muscle. With an average diameter of 20 µm, this corresponds to a surface area of 12 mm^2 per cubic millimeter of muscle. Perhaps only a few percent of the capillaries are open at any time, but there is still a considerable area for exchange of oxygen and carbon dioxide.

The driving force for gas exchange across the capillary wall is the difference in tension (partial pressure): the gas moves from a region of high partial pressure to a region of lower partial pressure. Thus, oxygen leaves the blood and passes into the tissue because the partial pressure (pO_2) is greater in the blood than in the tissue. Likewise, carbon dioxide passes from tissue into the blood because pCO_2 is greater in the tissue. In the lung, the pressure

TABLE 4.3   Sizes and Wall Stress in Blood Vessels

	P (torr)	R (cm)	T (dyne/cm)
Aorta	100	1.2	156,000
Artery	90	0.5	60,000
Capillary	30	0.0006	24
Vein	15	0.02	400
Vena cava	10	1.5	20,000

gradients are reversed. Oxygen and carbon dioxide exchange are discussed in Chapter 2.

Respiration

The respiratory center for nervous control of breathing is sensitive to the carbon dioxide tension and to blood pH: when the tension gets too high, the respiration rate or inhaled air volume is increased. The average respiration rate for the adult at rest is 14 breaths per minute, but the rate increases with exercise. With a tidal volume of 500 ml and dead space of 150 ml, hence a net volume of 350 ml, pulmonary ventilation is 14 × 500 ml, or 7 l/min, whereas alveolar ventilation is 14 × 350, or 5 l/min, approximately. With exercising, ventilation may be 10 times greater. The solubility of oxygen in tissue fluid is not great, but the alveolar surface area for gas exchange is about 75 m². The surface is divided among some 300 × 10⁶ alveoli, each about 0.2 mm in diameter with a wall 0.4 mm thick. The blood spends about 0.7 second in the alveolus (resting) or 0.3 second (exercising, with higher heart rate). This is sufficient to raise the oxygen tension of the blood to 100 percent of saturation.

The lungs are essentially passive in breathing; air is inhaled and exhaled as a result of changes in volume of the thoracic cavity (principally by flexing of the diaphragm) and concomitant variations in pressure in the airways. A patient with a narrowed or partially obstructed airway, which increases the flow resistance, has increased pressure and decreased flow rate. A mechanical respirator such as diagrammed in Fig. 4.14 may be used to pump air or oxygen into the lungs.

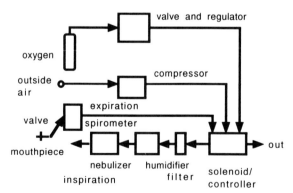

FIG. 4.14 Diagram of ventilator. Patient breathes in and out through mouth; valve selects path. Air, oxygen, or a mixture is supplied for inspiration, and water vapor is added. Filter removes bacteria. Expiration is through a spirometer. Pressure is regulated.

Heart Valve Prostheses

Replacement of diseased or defective heart valves by mechanical prostheses has been accomplished. Some types of artificial mitral (check) valves are illustrated in Fig. 4.15. These include the tilting disk, leaflet, and caged ball designs. The caged ball design is durable, minimizes hemolysis, and has the longest history of clinical use. Materials of construction include titanium, stellite 21 alloy, pyrolytic carbon, silicone rubber, and Dacron polyester cloth for attachment of the valve body to the heart tissue. Pyrolytic carbon and silicone rubber resist thrombus formation because the material becomes covered with protein, approximating tissue. Porcine valves are also used; they are treated with preservatives such as glutaraldehyde to reduce antigenicity and improve stability of the collagen.

Design considerations include reducing resistance to blood flow when the valve is open and minimizing back flow when it is closed, preventing mechanical hemolysis resulting from turbulence or excessive shear, using nonthrombogenic materials and preventing stasis, minimizing wear and fatigue and designing for a lifetime of 10 to 30 years, providing a simple and secure attachment method, and allowing for sterilization, noiseless operation, and

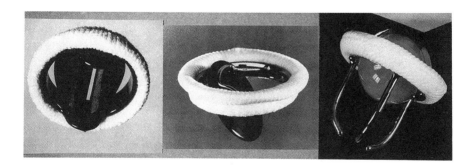

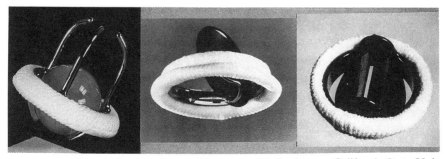

FIG. 4.15 Heart valve prostheses. (Courtesy of T. B. Davey, California State University, Sacramento).

operation in any position. Despite the thromboresistant design, at present it is necessary for the patient to receive anticoagulant agents indefinitely, to minimize thromboembolism.

Heart Assist and Artificial Heart

Replacements for the left ventricle, or for both ventricles and valves of the heart, have been developed for temporary use until a suitable human heart becomes available for transplant. A total artificial heart design is shown in Fig. 4.16. It consists of an inlet valve, a blood-pumping chamber with a power source, and an outlet valve, replacing the left and right ventricles and valves. The blood pump may be a balloon or diaphragm operated by an electric pump or compressed air, in synchronization with the heart cycle.

The total "permanent" artificial heart replacement is still not completely satisfactory, but has the advantage that patients do not have to be dependent on the limited supply of suitable donor hearts. The Jarvik heart, which has received most publicity, uses an external pump and a supply of compressed air to inflate or deflate an ellipsoidal sac that is alternately emptied and filled with blood. Unfortunately, the patient is then tethered to the air compressor.

Heart-Lung Machines

Heart bypass and oxygenator machines are used for surgery with the heart stopped and cooled. Figure 4.17 diagrams a type of cardiopulmonary bypass machine, one with a membrane oxygenator. Heart-lung machines also include pumps, a heat exchanger to chill the blood—and thus the body—filters, a bubble trap to eliminate any air emboli, and a blood reservoir. Parts are designed to minimize the amount of blood needed to fill or prime the machine. Roller pumps are used with a variable-speed rotating armature on large-diameter vinyl tubing filled with blood, so that the armature never contacts the blood (peristaltic pump). Despite careful design, hemolysis does occur and pumping should not continue beyond a few hours. Because erythrocytes contain ADP and erythrocytin, which promote clot formation, hemolysis is to be avoided. A thrombus may also form under conditions of turbulence or stasis, e.g., when the bloodstream encounters a projecting surface, bend, sudden contraction or expansion, or rough surfaces. Indwelling catheters are usually made of silicone rubber or another biocompatible polymer. All parts must be sterilizable, and some parts may be disposable to avoid resterilization.

Oxygenators are designed to oxygenate the blood and remove carbon dioxide with good efficiency. Oxygen addition should exceed carbon dioxide removal by approximately 30 percent to maintain physiological balance. Direct-contact oxygenators may be of the film or bubble type, or a combination. The film oxygenator allows venous blood to flow over a mesh or over a rotating, partially submerged cylinder or disk. The bubble oxygenator bubbles oxygen through venous blood; the blood then flows through a filter and trap

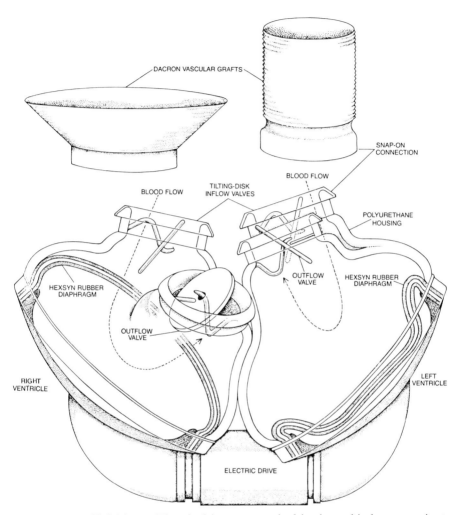

FIG. 4.16 Artificial heart. Electric drive; pneumatic drive is used in human patient hearts. Heart is sewed into natural atria and blood vessels with Dacron sleeves (Jarvik, R. K., 1981. The total artificial heart. *Sci. Am.* 244(1): 75.)

to remove bubbles. Cooling the blood helps to reduce oxygen emboli formation. Direct contact, however, tends to denature proteins and damage blood cells. Membrane oxygenators simulate the lung, using a thin semipermeable membrane to separate a film of blood and the oxygen. Artificial membranes are not as efficient as the natural membranes of the alveoli. Figure 4.18 is a diagram of a membrane oxygenator.

Gas exchange may be limited by high resistance to convective diffusion in blood or by high resistance to diffusion in the membrane as compared with diffusion in the blood, or reaction-limited if transport in membrane and fluid

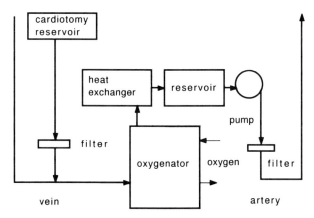

FIG. 4.17   Schematic of heart-lung machine.

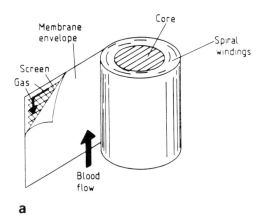

a

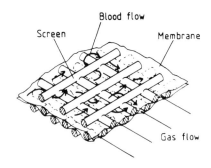

b

FIG. 4.18   Membrane oxygenator. Gaylor, J. D. S. 1988. Membrane oxygenators: Current developments in design and application. *J. Biomed. Eng.* 10: 542. By permission of publisher, Butterworth-Heineme.)

phases is very efficient. Assuming limiting by blood diffusion in a direct-contact oxygenator, with local equilibrium conditions, the mass of oxygen transferred across an element of area dS, in time t, is expressed as

$$dm/dS = (at/L)(P_i - P_b)D \text{ Nu}, \qquad (4.8)$$

where a = solubility of oxygen in blood = 0.3×10^{-4} ml(STP)/ml-torr
   P_i = partial pressure of oxygen at the interface, typically 700 torr in an oxygenator,
   P_b = partial pressure of oxygen in venous blood, typically 40 torr,
   D = diffusivity of oxygen in blood = 0.8×10^{-5} cm²/s,
   L = characteristic length (cm),
   Nu = local Nusselt number, hL/D (See Cook and Webster, listed in this chapter's Bibliography, for an expression).

In a membrane oxygenator using silicone rubber, the limiting condition is usually the mass transfer of carbon dioxide, as the oxygen transfer is more efficient. For an oxygenator element with two parallel plate membranes, the length (X) required to reduce the partial pressure of carbon dioxide in blood from P_0 to P_X is given as follows:

$$X = \frac{KQd}{2WDa} \ln \frac{P_0}{P_x}, \qquad (4.9)$$

where K = 2.5×10^{-4} mol/l torr
   Q = blood flow rate (ml/s)
   d = thickness of membrane (cm)
   W = width of plates (cm)
   D = permeability of membrane to CO_2 = 8.33×10^{-11} mol-cm/cm²-min-torr

A measure of efficiency is the ratio of total blood flow rate to priming volume (volume of blood in the oxygenator). For the lung, with a blood flow rate of 3000 1/min and a lung capillary volume of 100 ml, the efficiency is 30/min. For an oxygenator with 25 µm silicone rubber membrane thickness, the efficiency is about 12/min.

4.6   ARTIFICIAL KIDNEY

Renal Physiology

The functional unit of the kidney is the nephron, composed of (1) the glomerulus, a membrane or filter, (2) the proximal tubule, (3) the loop of Henle, and (4) the distal tubule. The hydrostatic pressure difference of about 70 torr between the afferent and efferent arterioles of the glomerulus causes the filtrate to cross the glomerulus into the proximal tubule. The filtrate is blood plasma less large protein molecules (mass greater than 30,000 daltons). The collective glomerular filtration rate is about 120 ml/min.

In passing along the proximal tubule, active and passive processes result in reabsorption of 65 to 76 percent of the water, nearly all electrolytes and crystalloids, and most of the amino acids, proteins, and polypeptides in the glomerular filtrate. The remaining fluid and solutes continue along the loop of Henle, the distal tubule, and into the renal pelvis and ureter. During the passage, the composition and concentration of solutes is altered compared to the arteriole by selective absorption, secretion, diffusion, and osmosis. The output is about 1.5 liters of urine per 24 hours. An example of the exchange is the sodium ion. Concentration of sodium in the glomerular filtrate is about the same as in plasma. In the proximal tubule, active (energy-requiring) processes result in reabsorption of 65 to 75 percent against the concentration gradient. Water follows the resulting osmolar gradient. Further adjustment takes place in the loop of Henle and the distal tubule as influenced by steroid hormones produced in the adrenal gland. Urea (protein breakdown product) is removed by glomerular filtration, but some is reabsorbed in the loop of Henle. Creatine (waste product of muscle metabolism) is removed by glomerular filtration. Uric acid (nucleic acid breakdown product) is secreted into the distal tubule from the tubular cells.

In addition to eliminating waste products and maintaining normal body water and electrolyte composition, the kidney also helps maintain the acid-base balance. An excess of hydrogen ions is produced by metabolic processes and ingested as protein. The kidney exchanges H^+ for Na^+ in the renal tubules and stabilizes pH by a carbon-dioxide/bicarbonate buffer, a hydrogen/dihydrogen phosphate buffer, and an ammonia/ammonium buffer. Ammonia is produced in the tubular cells from glutamate. The pH of normal urine is 5.0 to 6.5, and thus acidic.

The kidney is involved in synthesis of vitamin D, which assists in absorption of calcium from the gut and helps maintain skeletal homeostasis. The kidney also produces a precursor to erythropoietin, a hormone responsible for release of red blood cells from the marrow into the circulation.

Renal failure may result from trauma, blood loss, severe dehydration, burns, infection, toxic chemicals such as heavy metal compounds, disease such as diabetes mellitus, and other causes. In some cases, appropriate therapy allows the kidney to recover. If the damage is too severe, however, recourse is either a kidney transplant, an "artificial kidney," or dialysis machine. If a suitable donor kidney is not available, dialysis may be lifesaving, although artificial dialysis has its drawbacks and does not perform all of the functions of the natural kidney. For example, it may remove substances that the natural kidney recycles, and fails to remove some substances.

Dialysis Machines

The dialysis machine is a bioengineered substitute for the major functions of the natural kidney, designed to remove metabolic waste products, water, and other substances from the blood. Hemodialysis is the extracorporeal passage of blood through a semipermeable membrane that allows diffusion, and thus the removal of water and waste products. Peritoneal dialysis uses the peritoneum, a membrane lining the abdominal cavity, and instillation of fluid, electrolytes, and glucose to permit dialysis or diffusion of the waste products and removal of water by osmosis. Hemofiltration is extracorporeal circulation of blood along a membrane with application of hydrostatic pressure; the loss of fluid is overcome with intravenous infusion of saline. Hemoperfusion is passage of blood over an absorber (such as activated charcoal) or ion exchange resins that remove toxic products. The following discussion concentrates on hemodialysis.

A diagram of a typical hemodialysis machine is shown in Fig. 4.19. The major component is the dialyzer unit, which contains a semipermeable membrane (in a supporting structure), with blood pumped through one side and a physiologic dialysis solution or dialysate on the other. Various configurations of a dialyzer are pictured in Fig. 4.20. An arteriovenous shunt may be arranged with cannulas implanted surgically in the femoral artery and vein; during dialysis the silicone rubber shunt tubing is instead connected to the machine. Another approach is an arteriovenous fistula, in which an artery is connected directly to a vein, distending it and allowing connections to be made with large-bore needles. The machine itself has pumps, valves, gauges, and a heater in addition to the dialyzer.

Hemodialysis is usually performed three times weekly. The treatments are usually carried out for 3 to 6 hours, enough to clear urea from at least 120 liters of blood per week, as compared with a clearance rate of 1200 l/week for the natural kidneys. Because of the intermittent nature of the dialysis and the inefficiency of the artificial kidney, the urea level is variable and high,

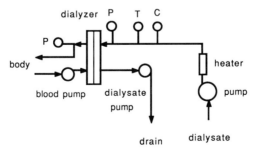

FIG. 4.19 Principle of hemodialysis machine. P = pressure gage; T = temperature sensor, C = conductivity meter.

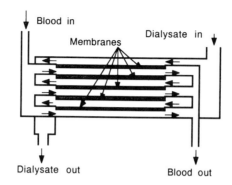

(a) Principle of flat membrane dialyzer

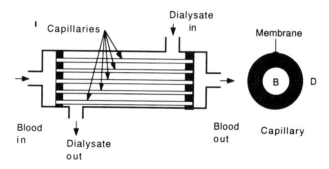

(b) Principle of capillary bundle dialyzer

FIG. 4.20 Dialyzer designs: flat parallel plate and capillary tube bundle (disposable).

some 14 to 200 mg/100 ml of blood, as compared with a normal 20 to 40 mg/ 100 ml. Standard cellulose membranes freely pass low molecular weight molecules such as urea, creatine, uric acid, and electrolytes, but are inefficient in removing high molecular weight molecules (of more than 200 daltons) and some toxins. The membranes pass, and therefore remove without reabsorption, amino acids, vitamins, glucose, and many other substances, as well as water. While many substances can be replaced by intravenous infusion, some are expensive and others may not even be known. In addition to the problem of removing certain substances while maintaining the concentrations of others, the cost of dialysis equipment, services, etc., results in a patient expense of $10,000 to $25,000 per year.

In a dialyzer, blood flows between two membrane sheets or inside a hollow fiber, while dialysate flows either concurrently or countercurrently on the outside of the membrane. Water removal can be predicted from the following equation:

$$Q = AL(\Delta P - \Delta p), \tag{4.10}$$

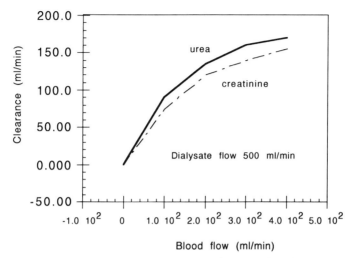

FIG. 4.21   Clearance vs. blood flow for dialysis.

where Q is the water (ml) removed per hour, A is the area (m^2) of the membrane, L (ml/[h-m^2-torr]) is the ultrafiltration index of the membrane (typically 3 to 15), ΔP (torr) is the mean hydrostatic pressure difference across the membrane, and Δp (torr) is the osmotic pressure of the proteins (25 torr). ΔP is determined by the required water removal rate and may be about 140 torr.

The solute removal rate or clearance rate C (ml/min) may be obtained from experimental data and fit to the expression

$$C = a_0 + a_1 Q_V + a_2 \frac{1}{Q_B}, \qquad (4.11)$$

where a_0, a_1, and a_2 are experimentally determined coefficients, Q_V is the ultrafiltration rate and Q_B is blood flow rate. Figure 4.21 illustrates the clearance rate of two substances as a function of blood flow rate and fixed dialysate flow rate, for a specific membrane, of a 1.1 m^2 area. The ultrafiltration index, L, of membranes varies from 1.5 to 30 ml/h-m^2-torr.

4.7   THERMAL MODELS

Internal Sources

The body obtains energy from the oxidation of food and from external sources of heat. Aside from about 5 percent of the food energy excreted in the feces and urine, the chemical energy derived from food is converted into products and processes in the cells, aids in maintaining a constant body temperature, and allows the performance of mechanical work by the muscles. Any energy in excess of the body's immediate requirements is stored as fat. Conversely, body fat is consumed when the caloric value of the food intake is less than the energy consumed in performing mechanical work and maintaining the body temperature. (When the fat is used up, the body begins to use muscle for heat energy.) Excess heat is removed by forced convection of the blood by the heart. Some heat is lost through the respiratory system by warming and humidification of exhaled air, but the major heat loss is through the skin. The temperature of the body core is sensed by a center in the hypothalamus, acting as a thermostat with a set point of 37°C. Heat loss from the skin can be increased by shunting and vasodilation of the arterioles so that more blood flows to the skin; conversely, heat is conserved by limiting blood flow to the skin by vasoconstriction. Another source of heat loss is evaporation of sweat, and the amount of sweat produced is regulated by the hypothalamus. The distribution of the hair, acting as an insulator, provides additional control, as do clothing and fat insulation. If necessary, more heat can be generated by muscular activity including shivering.

The basal metabolic rate (BMR), or energy requirement at rest, varies with species and individual characteristics, including sex, age, height, and weight (or, more closely, with skin area because heat is lost through the skin). In the adult human male, with a standard skin area of 1.85 m^2, the BMR is about 92 kcal/h = 92 C/h = 107 W. The BMR is regulated by thyroid hormone; hyperthyroid individuals have a higher BMR and hypothyroid persons have a lower BMR than euthyroid (normal) persons. Another variable affecting BMR is body temperature, because biochemical reactions are quite temperature dependent. An increase of 1°C increases the metabolic rate by 10 percent. Normal body temperature is 37°C. Typically, 25 percent of the BMR is used by the heart and other muscles, 19 percent by the brain, 10 percent by the kidneys, and 27 percent by the liver and spleen. Exercise, of course, consumes energy and causes the metabolic rate to increase above the BMR.

In isometric contraction, all of the energy applied to the muscle appears as heat. In isotonic contraction, the rate of performing work is the power product of F & v, where F is the force exerted and v is the velocity. The efficiency varies from 3 to 20 percent, depending on the type of activity; the rest appears as heat.

Heat Removal

The rate of heat production for a 2500 kcal/day diet, assuming no change in weight, is about 1.7 kcal/min or 120 W. To maintain a constant body temperature, heat must be lost at the same rate. The most important heat loss processes are radiation, convection, evaporation of sweat from the skin, and respiration. The actual heat loss depends on the temperature of the environment, humidity, wind speed, and insulation. The radiant heat transfer, for small differences in temperature, is given approximately as

$$H_r = K_r A \varepsilon (T_s - T_w), \tag{4.12}$$

where K_r is about 5.0 kcal/m^2 h °C, A is the skin area radiating, ε is the emissivity (nearly equal to 1), T_s is the skin temperature (°C), and T_w is the temperature of the surrounding walls. For a nude body of 1.2 m^2 surface area and skin temperature of 34°C, with walls at 25°C, the heat radiated is 54 kcal/h, or about 54 percent of the total rate of heat loss.

The heat loss by air convection past the nude body is given as

$$H_c = K_c A (T_s - T_a), \tag{4.13}$$

where T_a is the air temperature and K_c is the convection coefficient, a function of wind speed (or relative motion of body and air). For zero wind speed, $K_c = 2.3$ kcal/m^2 h °C. For a 1.2 m^2 area, 34°C skin temperature, and 25°C air temperature, the heat loss by convection is about 25 kcal/h, or about 25 percent of the body's heat loss rate.

Evaporation of sweat from the body at rest amounts to about 7 kcal/h, or 7 percent of the heat loss. Respiration adds another 14 kcal/h, or 14 percent of the total. When the skin is too hot and sweating increases, the latent heat of evaporation is removed, 580 kcal/l. In a hot climate or with vigorous exercise, a man may sweat at least 1 liter per hour.

External Source and Tissue Model

Models and data on the thermal properties of tissue, including the effect of blood perfusion, are discussed by Chato in the *Handbook of Bioengineering*, listed in this chapter's Bibliography, with references to more complete publications.

The time-dependent Pennes bioheat equation (expressed for one-dimensional geometry) is as follows:

$$\rho c (dT/dt) = \kappa (d^2 T/dx^2) + w c_b (T_a - T_v) + q, \tag{4.14}$$

where T is the tissue temperature, T_a is the local arterial or blood supply temperature, T_v is the local venous or tissue temperature, c_b is the specific heat of blood (about 3.7 kJ/kg °C), c is the specific heat of tissue (about equal that of blood), ρ is the tissue density (about 1030 kg/m^3), w is the blood perfusion rate (volume of perfused blood per volume of tissue, per unit time), and q is the volumetric heat generation rate. The thermal conductivity (κ) is 0.4 to 0.6 (W/m °C), depending on the tissue. This equation, solved subject to boundary conditions, gives the temperature as a function of position. It

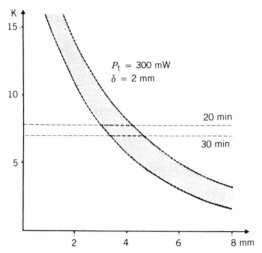

FIG. 4.22 Steady-state temperature rise vs. distance from fiber end. The upper and lower bounds of the shaded region correspond to low blood flow (δ_v = 10 mm) to medium blood flow (δ_v = 5 mm). Optical power P = 300 mW, optical penetration depth δ = 2 mm. (Svaasand, L. O. 1984. Dosimetry for photoradiation therapy. In *Porphyrins in tumor phototherapy*, ed. A. Andreoni and R. Cubbedu. New York: Plenum Publishing.)

may be used for steady-state heating with electromagnetic fields or ultrasound (hyperthermia), or for absorption of optical energy as in laser surgery.

Expressed in three dimensions, and for optical heating, the thermal balance can be rewritten as

$$\nabla T - \frac{1}{\alpha}\frac{\partial T}{\partial t} - \frac{T}{\delta_v^2} = -\frac{\beta\phi}{\kappa}, \tag{4.15}$$

where T is measured relative to the arterial temperature as zero, the thermal diffusivity

$$\alpha = \kappa/\rho c \tag{4.16}$$

the specific heat of tissue and blood are assumed to be the same, and the thermal penetration depth

$$\delta_v = \sqrt{\alpha/w}, \tag{4.17}$$

β is the rate of heat absorption from the light, per unit energy fluence density (ϕ). A correction is needed if heat is lost by radiation and convection at a surface, or removed by blood.

The steady-state temperature rise from a spherical emitter of power (P)

and radius (a) embedded in vascular tissue, with optical penetration depth (δ) (*e*-folding length for exponential attenuation of the light versus distance from the emitter) is then

$$T = \frac{P}{4\pi\kappa\left(1 - \left(\dfrac{\delta}{\delta_v}\right)^2\right)r}\left\{\frac{e^{-\dfrac{r-a}{\delta_v}}}{1 + \dfrac{a}{\delta_v}} - \frac{e^{-\dfrac{r-a}{\delta}}}{1 + \dfrac{a}{\delta}}\right\} \qquad (4.18)$$

An example is plotted in Fig. 4.22.

4.8 DRUG DELIVERY

Drugs may be delivered by oral administration, by injection (hypodermically, intramuscularly), or through the skin or lung. Once in the blood plasma, a drug may be metabolized or excreted, resulting in a time-dependent dose rate, as illustrated in Fig. 4.23. Usually, a constant drug concentration is desired for maximum effect. This may be achieved by constant infusion of the drug. For example, the drug may be dissolved in water in a collapsible bag, with an adjustable valve to control the rate of drop formation. The drops then flow through tubing to a cannula, which is inserted intravenously.

An alternative method is time-release of the drug from a polymer matrix or microcapsule, internally or through the skin, as indicated in Fig. 4.24.

The ideal would be an implantable sensor for the variable to be controlled, an implantable reservoir and pump (or equivalent), and a control device. For

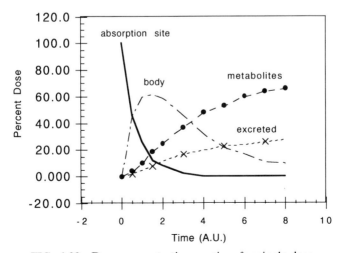

FIG. 4.23 Drug concentration vs. time for single dose.

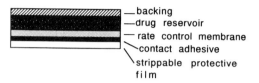

(a) Single sided patch

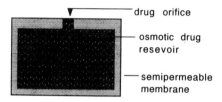

(b) Drug delivery by osmotic pressure
of water

FIG. 4.24 Drug delivery with rate controlled by polymeric membrane.

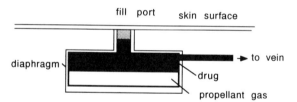

FIG. 4.25 Implantable drug delivery pump.

example, in diabetes mellitus, the blood glucose level varies with diet and exercise. Glucose sensor has been developed, using the sensing method discussed in Chapter 3. An implantable drug chamber with propellant is shown in Fig. 4.25. A similar chamber might be used in an implanted insulin delivery system for patients.

BIBLIOGRAPHY

Black, J. 1981. *Biological performance of materials: Fundamentals of biocompatibility*. New York: Marcel Dekker.

Cameron, J. G., and J. G. Skofronick. 1978. *Medical physics*. New York: John Wiley & Sons.

Cook, A. M., and J. G. Webster. 1982. *Therapeutic medical devices: Application and design*. Englewood Cliffs, N.J.: Prentice-Hall.

Florence, A. T., and D. Attwood. 1988. *Physicochemical principles of pharmacy*. 2d ed. New York: Chapman and Hall.

Jarvik, R. K. 1981. The total artificial heart. *Scientific American* 244(1): 66–72.

Park, J. B. 1984. *Biomaterials science and engineering.* New York: Plenum Press.

Petrofsky, J. S., and C. A. Phillips. 1986. Closed loop control of movement of skeletal muscle. *CRC critical reviews in biomedical engineering* 13(1): 35–95.

Rowland, M., and T. N. Tozer. 1989. *Clinical pharmokinetics.* 2nd ed. Philadelphia: Lea & Febiger.

Skalak, R., and S. Chien, eds. 1987. *Handbook of bioengineering.* New York: McGraw-Hill.

Selkurt, E. E., 1966. *Physiology.* 2d ed. Boston: Little Brown.

Svaasand, L. O., 1984. Thermal and optical dosimetry for photoradiation therapy of malignant tumors. In *Porphyrins in tumor phototherapy*, ed. A. Andreoni and R. Cubeddu. New York: Plenum Press.

Vander, A. J., J. H. Sherman, and D. S. Luciano, 1970. *Human physiology: The mechanisms of body function.* New York: McGraw-Hill.

CHAPTER 5

LASERS AND OPTICS

5.0 LASERS AND OPTICS IN MEDICINE

Lasers are used for surgery, photodynamic therapy of cancer, and for diagnosis by fluorescence. Optics are used in many medical instruments.

5.1 LASERS

Laser is an acronym for *l*ight *a*mplification by *s*timulated *e*mission of *r*adiation. An essential attribute of any laser is stimulated emission in an active material (except for the free electron laser, which uses an electron beam in a vacuum).

Stimulated Emission and Pumping

Most molecules (or atoms, or ions) of a material are in the lowest quantum energy state, the ground state. Because of thermal agitation, a few molecules are in excited states. For laser action, one must create a population inversion, in which more molecules are in excited states than in the ground state (at least for the energy levels involved in the laser transition). The process of adding energy to create a population inversion is called *pumping*. The most common forms of pumping are (1) optical and (2) electrical discharge or current (chemical and nuclear pumping are rare and are not used in medical lasers).

The principle of stimulated absorption of a light photon whose energy matches the energy between two levels of the molecule is shown in Fig. 5.1a. Spontaneous emission of a photon, in which the molecule randomly returns

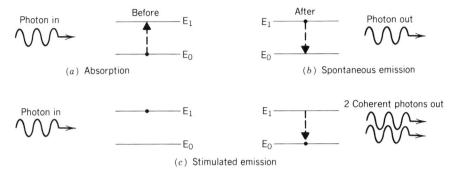

FIG. 5.1 (a) Absorption, (b) spontaneous emission, and (c) stimulated emission.

to ground-state energy (or at least a lower energy state) is illustrated in Fig. 5.1b. Stimulated emission of a photon (Fig. 5.1c) occurs when the molecule interacts with an incoming photon with energy equal to the molecular transition energy, resulting in emission of a photon of equal energy. In the wave picture, the frequency and phase of the stimulated emission is equal to the frequency and phase of the stimulating light wave (i.e., the waves are coherent).

Figure 5.2 illustrates the optical pumping of a three-level system, typical of doped insulator lasers. In this example, most atoms are in the ground state, E_0, with no pumping. With moderate pumping, atoms are raised to a metastable level E_2 by stimulated absorption. The level rapidly decays to level E_1. With intense pumping, e.g., from a xenon flash lamp, stimulated emission occurs with a photon energy of E_1 to E_0. The emitted light is monochromatic. Another method of pumping is to pass an electric current through the active material, e.g., a gas. The helium-neon neutral gas laser and the argon ion laser are of this type. The glass or other vessel is filled with the gas, and a cathode and anode are located within the vessel. A DC voltage is applied between the electrodes, generating an electrical discharge. These lasers are usually very inefficient, as only a small fraction (on the order of 0.1 percent) actually serves to pump the gas molecules or ions into a regime of population inversion.

Optical Feedback

Another requirement for a laser light amplifier (and oscillator) is optical feedback. This is normally achieved by making the active medium in the form of a long cylinder with a mirror on each end, arranged to reflect light back into the active medium along the axis of the cylinder, as seen in Fig. 5.3. The resulting combination of mirrors is called an *optical cavity* or *resonator*, analogous to the cavities of microwave oscillators and amplifiers. One mirror is made 100 percent reflective or nearly so. The other mirror is perhaps 97 to 98 percent reflective, allowing 2 to 3 percent of the light to escape as a beam.

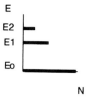

(a) No pumping

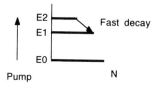

(b) Pumping below lasing threshold

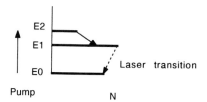

FIG. 5.2 Pumping of energy levels, population inversion, and laser transition.

(c) Higher pumping: laser action

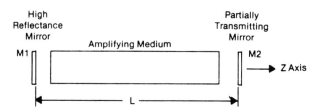

FIG. 5.3 Optical resonator with totally and partially reflecting mirrors.

Because of the geometry and repeated reflections before escape, the beam is collimated (parallel rays with divergence on the order of milliradians). Diode lasers do not use mirrors, but the material has a high refractive index, so that considerable reflection does occur at the surface or "facet"; the opposite facet is mirrored. The beam is irregular, as compared with the cylindrical beam of most other lasers, and special focusing or collimating optics are needed.

Plane mirrors are seldom used, because of the difficulty of alignment. Usually they are curved, e.g., concave. They may be built into the active material container or solid material itself, or may be located outside the region of active material. If outside, the light beam is transmitted through windows (e.g., polished, plane parallel glass) set at Brewster's angle of incidence for minimal reflectance (the light polarized in one direction is not reflected at all; the transmitted beam is then polarized). Brewster's angle is the arc tangent of the relative refractive index; for glass $(n_1/n_0) = 1.5$ and the Brewster angle is $56.5°$.

TEM Modes

The multiple reflections between the mirrors set up a standing wave pattern, which may be described in terms of longitudinal modes, but only a few of the many frequencies involved in the standing waves will be amplified. Of more general interest is the transverse mode structure, which describes how the electric and magnetic fields vary with the x and y (transverse) coordinates. These modes are described by TEM_{lm} (transverse electromagnetic field with the integer l giving the number of times the electric or magnetic field crosses the x axis, and m the number of times the electric or magnetic field crosses the y axis). The integers l and m are also the number of nodes (regions of little or no light) in the corresponding direction. If the laser beam is projected on a surface, one may see spots corresponding to the various TEM patterns. In medical and other applications, the TEM_{00} pattern is desirable, as shown in Fig. 5.4. The mirrors are aligned until this condition is met. The intensity (irradiance) distribution in the TEM_{00} mode is not uniform, but has a Gaussian distribution. This is important in defining spot size, or the radius of the laser beam. The standard nomenclature defines the spot or beam in terms of the radius w where the electric field strength falls to $1/e = 0.367$ of the peak strength, with a corresponding intensity (watts/m²) of $(0.367)^2 = 0.135$ of peak intensity.

Directionality

The optical resonator is also responsible for the directionality (collimation) of the laser beam. The light may make hundreds of reflections before finally being transmitted by the exit mirror. Each time the original source appears to be farther distant, whereas the wave front is collimated by the exit aperture or mirror. The full angle beam divergence is defined as twice the angle that the radius at 0.367 of the maximum amplitude makes with the center of the beam. It can be determined by measuring the beam radii at two distances from the laser. Typically, the full angle beam divergence is 1 or 2 milliradians (for 1 mrad, the spot size increases by 1 mm per meter along the axis).

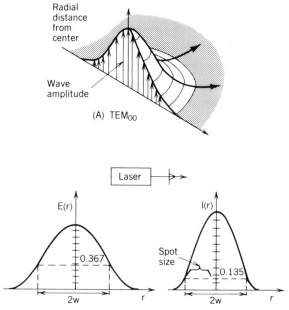

FIG. 5.4   Gaussian beam shape and electric field strength and intensity in TE_{00} mode laser beam.

Monochromaticity

Although laser light is nearly monochromatic, there is a very small spread in the frequency or wavelength for a single atomic energy transition because of Doppler or collisional broadening. This is so small (on the order of 0.1 percent) that it is often neglected. Light amplification may occur at more than one atomic transition, however. If only one wavelength (or a few closely spaced wavelengths) is desired, as is usually the case, the selection is made by special coatings on the mirrors, which are highly reflective only for a narrow band of wavelengths. The mirror or mirrors have to be changed to oscillate at other wavelengths. Often some adjustment (e.g., of gas discharge current, or of magnetic field) is made to enhance the emission from weak transitions. Very weak light (as compared with the laser beam) is emitted from the plasma discharge.

Coherence

The most unusual characteristic of a laser is the emission of coherent light, caused by the stimulated emission. Coherence means that the output waves are of the same frequency and phase and can interfere constructively or destructively in appropriate circumstances. Coherence is exploited in imaging by holography. Another aspect of coherence is the ability to focus to an extremely small spot size, limited by diffraction or aberrations of the lens. Waves can be spatially and/or temporally coherent. Spatial coherence describes the phase correlation of two different points across a wave front at a given instant; it is related to the apparent dimensions of the source (a point source is 100 percent spatially coherent). Temporal coherence describes the phase correlation of waves at a fixed point in space at two different times; it is related to the monochromaticity of the source (i.e., the more monochromatic, the more temporally coherent). If the phase difference between two points at different times is constant, the waves are both spatially and temporally coherent.

The degree of coherence can be obtained from an interference measurement, for example, in a double slit experiment. If the path difference between the wavelets from the two slits is equal to an odd number of half-wavelengths, the wavelets arrive at the screen 180° out of phase and interfere destructively, and a dark "fringe" appears. Likewise, constructive interference occurs and a bright fringe appears where the path difference is an even number of half-wavelengths. If coherence is less than 100 percent, the fringes are "washed out": the bright fringes are dimmer and the dark fringes are brighter. No fringes are seen, only an overall illumination, with an incoherent source. Effective coherence is achieved only over a limited region of space and time, even for a laser. The lateral coherence length is the lateral distance across a wave front for which the phase difference remains essentially constant (able to generate fringes). The longitudinal coherence length may be considered as the length of a wave train or wave packet over which the phase remains effectively constant (temporally coherent). The corresponding time, for which the wave is essentially monochromatic, is termed the *coherence time*.

Power and Radiance

Laser-beam power ranges from milliwatts to many watts. The power is limited by pumping power, heat transfer, and the inherent gain of the laser. Some types of lasers cannot achieve high powers with reasonable dimensions (e.g., the length of an optical resonator). Because of the small emitting area and divergence, a typical laser beam has a very high radiance (brightness), much higher than arc or incandescent lamps. For example, the radiance of a 1-watt laser with a beam area of 10^{-6} m^2 and solid angle of 10^{-6} steradian is 10^{12} W m^{-2} sr^{-1}.

Pulsing and Modulation

Lasers may be operated with steady power output (CW) or pulsed. A few lasers can be operated only in the pulsed mode. One way to pulse is to modulate the current in a gas discharge or similar electrically pumped laser, or the light in an optically pumped laser. Lasers that are pumped by xenon flash lamps are pulsed because the flash lamp is pulsed (typically with a pulse width on the order of a microsecond, and a low pulse repetition rate to allow for recharging the high voltage capacitors in the power supply). The beam can be pulsed (or otherwise modulated) by means of a mechanical chopper or a rotating mirror, or by electro-optic or acousto-optic shutters. The latter are often used for Q-switching. A transparent electro-optic crystal rotates the plane of polarization when a voltage is applied across it, and the beam is absorbed by a polarizer. An acousto-optic shutter works by diffracting the laser beam with sound waves (frequency 1 to 100 kHz), which change the refractive index of the medium, forming a three-dimensional grating. In another type of acousto-optic shutter, the sound wave is generated in a crystal and the beam is deflected through an angle to a slit.

The Q, or quality factor, of an electromagnetic cavity is the ratio of the energy stored (times 2π) to the energy dissipated per cycle. One method of obtaining short (less than 100 nanoseconds), intense (megawatts or so, peak power) pulses at relatively low repetition rates (single pulse to about 100 pulses/s) is to Q-switch. The idea is to switch from a lossy (low Q), nonlasing state while the population inversion is building, to a low-loss (high Q), lasing state. This can be done, for instance, by inserting an acousto-optic shutter in the laser cavity, arranged to deflect some of the beam from the cavity, thus creating a high loss. Then, at the instant of peak population inversion, the acoustic wave is shut off, the beam is undeflected, the medium rapidly builds to the lasing condition, and a pulse of light is emitted until the inverted population is depleted. Another way to Q-switch is to insert a dye cell, chosen so that the absorption of the dye decreases with irradiance, at the laser wavelength. There is an abrupt decrease in losses when the dye is bleached and thus no longer absorbing, and the Q switches from low to high values.

Mode locking is a method of obtaining extremely short pulses (few picoseconds), relatively high peak powers, and high repetition rates. Normally, a laser oscillates in many longitudinal modes, with random phases. Lasers can be forced into phase, and made to emit a very short pulse, if the loss in the laser cavity is varied at frequency c/2L, where c is the speed of light, and L is the cavity length. Thus, 2L/c is the round-trip time for a photon in the cavity. To mode lock, the shutter is opened for a very short time every 2L/c seconds and closed at other times. Passive mode locking can also be achieved with a saturable absorber (dye) in the cavity.

Types of Lasers

Table 5.1 gives the characteristics of some lasers, which are classified in the following list.

1. Gas lasers, pumped by an electrical discharge in a gas, such as the following:
   a. Neutral gas (e.g., helium-neon)
   b. Ion (argon and krypton)

c. Molecular gas (CO_2)
d. Metal vapor (e.g., helium-cadmium)
e. Excimer (e.g., KrF, XeCl)
2. Solid-state lasers, pumped by flash lamps
    a. Neodymium: YAG (yttrium aluminum garnet)
    b. Neodymium: glass
3. Semiconductor (diode) lasers
    a. GaAs and others
4. Dye lasers
    a. Dye solution, flash lamp pumped
    b. Dye solution, laser pumped
5. Free electron laser

Of these, probably the most commonly used are the carbon dioxide and neodymium lasers for surgery, and the argon laser for hemostasis (blood vessel coagulation). The UV excimer laser is currently used in laser surgery, exploiting a photoablative process rather than heat. The argon-laser–pumped dye laser is used in photodynamic therapy with hematoporphyrin-derivative, and a yellow dye laser in treatment of port wine birthmarks. Semiconductor (diode) lasers offer future promise although they are presently limited to wavelengths greater than 650 nm. So far the free electron laser (FEL) is not used in medicine, but its tunability in wavelength may allow its substitution for other lasers.

The construction of an ion laser "plasma tube" is indicated in Fig. 5.5. The filling gas may be argon (emitting at 488.0 and 514.5 nm), or krypton

TABLE 5.1 **Typical Laser Parameters**

Name	Wavelength (nm)	Power (W)	Divergence (mrad)	Pulse Width	Repetition Rate (Hz)
Nitrogen	337	300 peak	1×7	10 ns	1–50
Argon	458–514	5	0.5	CW	
Krypton	413	1	0.5	CW	
HeNe	633	0.01	1.0	CW	
CO_2	10,600	300	1.0	CW	
		2000	1.0	1 ms	1000
Excimer (XeCl)	308	100 mJ/pulse	N/A	100 ns	0–100
Nd:glass	1,060	8 J/pulse	5.0	1 ms	5
Nd:YAG	1,060	1	2.0	CW	
Diode	904	20 peak	large	0.1 μs	5000
Dye	430–780	1	N/A	CW pulsed if flash lamp pumped	

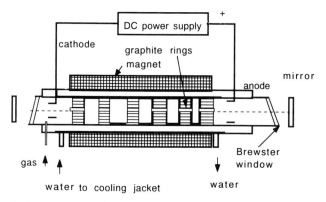

FIG. 5.5 Ion laser (e.g., Ar^+, Kr^+) with electrical excitation.

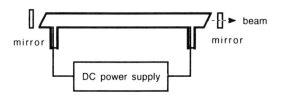

FIG. 5.6 Sealed-tube carbon dioxide laser. May also use axial or transverse gas flow and transverse excitation.

(647.1 nm, or with proper mirrors, in the UV range, at 413.1 nm). A water jacket and magnet surround the plasma tube.

Figure 5.6 shows a sealed carbon dioxide laser such as is used in laser surgery. The filling gas is typically 10 percent CO_2, 10 percent N_2, and the rest helium. The emission is centered around 10.6 μm. The tube may be sealed, or the gas may flow down or across the tube. If the tube is sealed, life is prolonged by adding H_2 or H_2O to the gas mixture, or by including a heated nickel catalyst, for recombination. Excitation is by DC discharge or by transverse RF. The sealed laser is capable of about 100 W, which is sufficient for laser surgery. Similar arrangements may be used in excimer lasers, which uses gases such as XeF and emit in the UV range (350 nm for XeF).

The arrangement of a flash lamp pumped laser (e.g., for a solid crystal or glass rod) is shown in Fig. 5.7. The Nd:YAG and Nd:glass lasers emit at about 1060 nm. The crystal or glass rod may be a few millimeters in diameter and a few centimeters long and is usually situated at one focus of a cylindrical, elliptical mirror, with the flash lamp at the other focus.

A semiconductor diode laser is shown schematically in Fig. 5.8. The rear cleaved surface may be mirrored. By changing the composition, different wavelengths can be obtained, so far from about 630 nm to 1000 nm. Powers

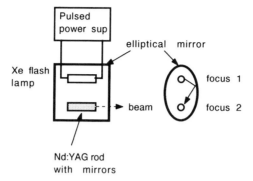

FIG. 5.7 Flash-lamp-pumped neodymium-doped yttrium-aluminum-garnet (Nd:YAG) laser.

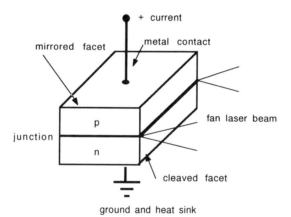

FIG. 5.8 Semiconductor diode laser. The semiconductor may be GaAs, for example.

over 1 W can be achieved. These lasers are much more efficient and smaller than gas or other types of lasers.

Figure 5.9 illustrates a laser-pumped dye laser. The dye laser can be tuned over a limited range of wavelengths using a suitable grating, prism, or etalon, but for a wider range it is necessary to change the dye. Dyes are best suited for the visible range. The pumping wavelength has to be shorter than the laser emission wavelength; dye lasers may be pumped with a broadband xenon flash lamp, nitrogen laser, or argon laser, depending on the emission desired.

Figure 5.10 diagrams an entirely different kind of laser, the FEL. A high voltage (MeV) electron beam travels down a vacuum pipe, equipped with mirrors for an optical resonator. The electron beam is deflected in a sinuous path by an array of magnets, the "wiggler" or "undulator." This causes emission of light, which is amplified by feedback between the light beam in the resonator and the electron beam. Present FELs are pulsed at a low

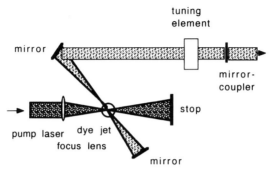

FIG. 5.9   Laser-pumped dye laser. Dye is in cell or jet perpendicular to page, from recirculation system.

repetition rate, limited by the electron accelerator. FELs are designed for operation in the infrared and visible spectrum. A significant advantage of an FEL is tunability over a wide range of wavelengths by varying the electron beam energy.

5.2   LENSES AND MIRRORS

Lenses and mirrors are used to form an image of an object. Even when the purpose is to transfer energy, one can consider using a lens or mirror forming an image of the laser beam, lamp filament, arc, or other source of light. When transferring energy, the image can be imperfect (just a blur spot).

Simple Lens

Figure 5.11 shows a simple, thin lens. The surfaces are segments of a sphere, and the light rays are paraxial (they lie so close to the optical axis that sines can be replaced by the angle itself). In the treatment that follows, the diameter and wavelength are such that diffraction may be neglected. It is also assumed that the lens is in air. A more complete treatment, including the refractive index and radius of curvature of the lens surface, is given, for example, in Hecht and Zajac (pp. 100–116), listed in the Bibliography at the end of this chapter. Figure 5.11 illustrates a double convex lens (positive or converging, with the center thicker than the edge). A lens may also be concave (negative or diverging, with the edge thicker than the center). The image focal length f_i is equal to the image distance s_i when the incident beam is parallel, and the object focal length f_o is the object distance s_o when the lens collimates the beam. For a thin lens, $f_o = f_i = f$ and is specified by the manufacturer.

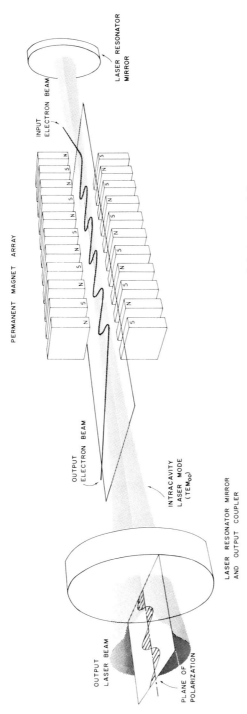

PERMANENT MAGNET ARRAY

INPUT ELECTRON BEAM

LASER RESONATOR MIRROR

OUTPUT ELECTRON BEAM

INTRACAVITY LASER MODE (TEM$_{00}$)

LASER RESONATOR MIRROR AND OUTPUT COUPLER

OUTPUT LASER BEAM

PLANE OF POLARIZATION

FIG. 5.10 Basic components of a free electron laser. The laser light is emitted from an accelerator electron beam, which is made to undulate by an array of permanent magnets. (Courtesy of L. Elias, University of California, Santa Barbara.)

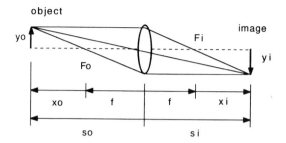

FIG. 5.11   Raytracing for simple, thin lens; o, object; i, image; f, focal length.

The relationship between the object distance s_o and the image distance s_i is given by the Gaussian lens formula

$$\frac{1}{s_o} + \frac{1}{s_i} = \frac{1}{f} \tag{5.1}$$

or the Newtonian form

$$x_o x_i = f^2. \tag{5.2}$$

The sign convention is as follows:

s_o and x_o are positive if to the left of the lens
s_i and x_i are positive if to the right of the lens
f is positive if converging, and negative if diverging

As an example, assume $f = 100$ mm and $s_o = 600$ mm, hence $s_i = 120$ mm. The transverse magnification M_T, or just magnification, and image of the object can be found by raytracing. One ray passes through the axis without deviation. A second ray is parallel to the optical axis and then passes through point F_i. A third ray passes through point F_o and is then refracted to become parallel to the axis. The transverse magnification is

$$M_T = \frac{y_i}{y_o} = -\frac{s_i}{s_o} \tag{5.3}$$

The longitudinal magnification is

$$M_L = \frac{-f^2}{x_o^2} = -M_{T^2} \tag{5.4}$$

The sign convention is

Positive s indicates a real object or image.

Positive y_o indicates an erect object, $+y_i$ an erect image.

Positive M_T indicates an erect image.

In the example discussed previously, $M_T = -120$ mm/600 mm $= -0.2$. The negative sign indicates an inverted image. For certain s_o, Table 5.2 lists the type of image, span of s_i, image orientation, and relative size.

A simple lens focuses to $s_i = f$, that is, the image distance is equal to the focal length if the incoming beam is collimated (object at infinity or at least far distant). If the beam is not collimated, the closest separation of the image and object occurs when each are at twice the focal length. Two lenses may be used to magnify or minify the image. The object is located at the focal length of the first lens, f_1. This collimates the beam. The second lens may be separated from the first by any convenient distance. The image is then located at the focal length of the second lens, f_2. The transverse magnification $M_T = s_i/s_o$. The general case of the compound lens, where two lenses at a certain separation and different focal lengths, is discussed by Hecht and Zajac, listed in this chapter's Bibliography.

Laser Focusing. The beam from a convex lens first converges to a spot in the focal plane and then diverges again. The smallest blur spot, in the focal plane, is set by diffraction

$$d = \frac{2.44\lambda s}{D} \tag{5.5}$$

approximately, where d is the diameter of the blur spot, λ is the wavelength of the light, D is the diameter of a collimated beam (which should be at least

TABLE 5.2 Properties of Simple Thin Lens

		Convex		
s_o	Image	s_i	Orientation	Size
∞ to 2f	real	f to 2f	inverted	minified
2f	real	2f	inverted	same
f to 2f	real	∞ to 2f	inverted	magnified
f		$+ - \infty$		
<f	virtual	$|s_i| > s_o$	erect	magnified
		Concave		
any	virtual	$|s_i| < |f|$	erect	minified

three times the beam diameter at the lens), and s is the working distance. The spot contains at least 80 percent of the power in a TE_{00} mode. Usually, the focal spot size is much larger, even when lens aberrations are negligible (as achieved with a well-corrected achromat).

When focusing an extended source with a lens at a large distance, it is convenient to consider the angle of divergence (θ) subtended by the source at the lens, neglecting aberrations and diffraction. Then

$$d = f\theta, \tag{5.6}$$

where d is the diameter of the blur spot and f is the focal length. For a laser, θ is the divergence of the beam. Thus, to obtain a small diameter spot, a short-focal-length lens should be used.

Fiberoptics is treated in the next section. However, for the present discussion it is sufficient to know that the diameter of the fiber is D and the divergence is θ. Then, for a convex lens, the simple thin lens formula applies, and the focal spot diameter d is given by

$$d = \frac{s_i D}{s_o} \tag{5.7}$$

The lens diameter has no effect on the size of the blur spot, but must equal at least $s_o\theta$ to capture all of the light emitted by the fiber.

The lens can focus the light emitted by the fiber to a very small diameter. If no lens is used, the spot diameter

$$d = D + l\theta, \tag{5.8}$$

where l is the distance from the end of the fiber to the tissue and θ is the divergence of the emitted light in radians.

Numerical Aperture

The numerical aperture (NA) of a lens is defined as the sine of the angle the marginal ray (at edge of lens, usually) makes with the optical axis. The NA on the object side of the lens of clear diameter D is

$$NA_o = \sin \theta_o = \frac{D}{2s_o}, \tag{5.9a}$$

whereas for the NA on the image side

$$NA_i = \sin \theta_i = \frac{D}{2s_i}. \tag{5.9b}$$

The $f/\#$ is f/D, and for small angles

$$f/\# = 1/2 \ NA \tag{5.10}$$

and is written as f/4, for example. If a laser beam is employed, the beam diameter is small and NA and f/# are not significant.

Thick Lens

The thin lens formulas can be used if the focal length (f) is replaced by the front focal length (f_f) (distance from the front focal point to the primary or front vertex of the lens) and the back focal length (f_b) (distance from the secondary or back vertex to the rear focal point). These specifications will normally be given by the manufacturer.

Aberrations. The focal length of a lens depends on the wavelength because of the variation of its refractive index, $n(\lambda)$. In the visible, the refractive index decreases with λ, f increases, and blue is focused closer to the lens than red. The axial distance between two such focal points is the axial chromatic aberration, ACA. One can remove chromatic aberration with a special compound lens, an achromatic doublet or achromat. A net focusing achromat consists of a convex lens of "crown" glass followed by a concave lens of "flint" glass in contact, often cemented together. The combination of simple lenses and glasses is chosen to remove the dispersion in wavelength (chromatic aberration) while still obtaining a net positive focal length. Glasses are specified in terms of the refractive index and the dispersive index, Abbe number, or V number, where

$$V_y = \frac{n_y - 1}{n_b - n_r}, \tag{5.11}$$

where y is a yellow wavelength (587.6 nm), b a blue wavelength (486.1 nm), and r a red wavelength (656.3 nm). The focal length of the achromat is specified at the yellow wavelength. Glasses with $n_y > 1.60$, $V_y > 50$, and $n_y < 1.60$, $V_y > 55$, are known as *crowns* and the others are known as *flints*. BK-7 is a crown (K = crown). Originally composed of borosilicates and other light element silicates, newer optical glasses contain rare earth elements such as lanthanum.

There are other aberrations, even for monochromatic light:

1. Spherical aberration
2. Coma
3. Astigmatism
4. Field curvature
5. Distortion

It is easiest to make lenses with spherical surfaces. However, these exhibit spherical aberration, in which rays refracted at greater radii are focused closer to the lens. It can be reduced by limiting the off-axis radius (f/2 or greater), by selecting the lens shape (planoconvex for distant objects, biconvex for equal or nearly equal object and image distances), by orienting the lens properly (most strongly curved surface toward a distant object), and by using a combination of converging and diverging lenses as in an achromat. If the lens is "faster" than f/2 (smaller f number) an aspheric lens may be needed, but this requires expensive special grinding and polishing procedures.

Coma is an aberration associated with an object point off-axis. It comes about because the "principal planes" are actually not planes, but curved surfaces. The magnification varies with the distance off-axis. The image has a tail like a comet, hence the name. Coma depends on the shape of the lens. The biconvex lens has zero coma. Coma can also be reduced by a proper stop (aperture).

Astigmatism occurs when the rays from an off-axis object point strike the lens asymmetrically. It increases as the object point moves more off-axis and the rays striking the lens become more oblique. The magnitude of the astigmatism aberration depends on the power of the lens and the angle with which the rays intersect the lens surface. It is mitigated by making the displacement of object points off-axis small.

Field curvature occurs because the focal surface is actually paraboloidal rather than plane. The eye can accommodate to moderate field curvature, and some cameras actually operate with a matching curved photosensitive surface. It is possible to cancel the positive field curvature of one lens by the negative field curvature of another lens. Some cameras are provided with a negative "field flattener" lens near the focal surface to cancel the field curvature of a positive lens.

Distortion occurs if the transverse magnification depends on the off-axis image point distance. For positive, or pincushion, distortion, the magnification is larger at greater distances. In negative, or barrel, distortion, magnification decreases with increasing distance. Thus the shape of objects is distorted in the image, even though the image is in focus. Distortion can be minimized by locating a stop between a combination of lenses.

Mirrors

Light does not traverse a mirror, and mirrors have zero chromatic aberration. Thus they can be used over a greater wavelength span than a lens. A mirror is often vacuum-evaporated aluminum on a highly polished metal or glass substrate. Reflection from the first surface produces an image (second-surface reflection occurs from metal behind glass, as in an ordinary mirror). The optics of mirrors can be derived from Snell's law, in which the angle of incidence, θ_i (measured from the normal to the surface), equals the angle of reflection, θ_r.

Plane Mirror. If reflected rays are extrapolated to the right of a mirror, one finds $|s_i| = |s_o|$. By convention, the signs are chosen so that s_i and s_o are negative when the object and image points are to the right of the mirror. This gives a formula for the image that is the same as the Gaussian lens equation (Eq. 5.1). The transverse magnification $M_T = +1$, and the image is the same size as the object, erect, and virtual. One cannot focus light into the image space, but the image can be viewed from the source side of the mirror. The image is reverted; that is, a right-handed coordinate system in the object space is converted to a left-handed coordinate system in the image space. For a symmetrical object, an odd number of reflections from planar mirrors will revert left for right, whereas an even number of reflections will give the correct orientation again. If the planar mirror is mounted on an axis and rotated through angle α, the reflected beam or image will rotate through 2α. Such mirrors are often used in laser-beam scanning.

Plane mirrors do not exhibit spherical aberration, coma, astigmatism, field curvature, or distortion.

If a mirror is only partially reflective, some of the light will be transmitted and some reflected. This is a beamsplitter, which can be used to divide or recombine a beam. If the thickness and material of the coating are correctly chosen, the beamsplitter is dichroic. (That is, it mostly transmits over a certain wavelength band and mostly reflects over an adjacent wavelength band. What is not transmitted is reflected in a different direction.)

Curved Mirrors. A concave spheroidal mirror focuses light, but has the same aberrations as lenses (with the exception of chromatic aberration). A concave mirror with a parabola as a cross section focuses an incident ray parallel to the optical axis (object at infinity) to a focal point on the axis, P. Conversely, light emitted at P is reflected into a ray parallel to the optical axis. The diameter of the mirror determines the energy received or emitted. The focal length is the distance from P to the vertex (point of mirror on axis). The paraboloidal mirror eliminates spherical aberration for the infinitely distant object point, but exhibits coma and astigmatism for off-axis points, restricting the paraboloidal mirror to large f/numbers and a narrow field of view.

The cross section of an ellipsoidal mirror is an ellipse. Light emitted at one focus is imaged at the other focus. The size of the mirror is based on the dimensions of the source, or perhaps the heat loading of the wall.

5.3   FIBEROPTICS

The principle of fiberoptic light transmission is total internal reflection. A typical light ray will be reflected thousands of times in traversing the fiber, but because of the low loss at each reflection, overall attenuation is relatively small. Consider the ray shown entering the polished end of a long cylindrical fiber of transparent material of low absorption glass, fused silica, liquid, or the like, as shown in Fig. 5.12. The fiberguide core has a refractive index of n_1 and is surrounded by a cladding of lower refractive index, n_2 (e.g., a plastic

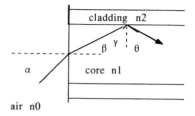

FIG. 5.12 Raytracing in a step-index fiber-optic lightguide. The refractive index of the cladding, n_2, is smaller than the index of the core, n_1.

or different glass). By Snell's law,

$$n_0 \sin \alpha = n_1 \sin \beta \qquad (5.12)$$

and the oblique ray is refracted toward the normal, because $n_1 > n_0$. The ray usually enters from air, which has a refractive index $n_0 = 1.000$. When the ray is incident on the core-cladding interface at angle $\gamma = (\pi/2) - \beta$, it is refracted by Snell's law to a different angle θ,

$$n_1 \sin \gamma = n_2 \sin \theta. \qquad (5.13)$$

For small α, θ is greater than $\pi/2$ and the ray is refracted back into the core, a process called *total internal reflection*. As α increases, so does θ, and at the critical angle $\theta_c = \pi/2$, the ray just remains in the core. At larger α, the ray is refracted but escapes from the core into the cladding and is no longer transmitted down the length of the fiber core. The critical angle is related to the refractive indexes of core and cladding. Referred to the incident angle,

$$n_o \sin \alpha = (n_1^2 - n_2^2)^{0.5}. \qquad (5.14)$$

A typical step-index fiber core glass has $n_1 = 1.62$, and cladding $n_2 = 1.52$.

Energy Transfer

Light collection by a fiber is proportional to the clear area of the core, A_c, and the acceptance angle α. The NA is a measure of the acceptance cone. The light-gathering power of the fiber can also be expressed in terms of the f number:

$$f/ = \frac{1}{(2 \tan \alpha)}. \qquad (5.15)$$

The cutoff with angle is not sharp because of off-axis and skew rays; instead one commonly finds a near Gaussian distribution with radius at the exit of the fiberguide, with a maximum of $\alpha = 0$, approaching zero at the critical angle given by equation 5.14.

The fiberguide core diameter may be on the order of 10 μm to 1000 μm and still be reasonably transmissive and mechanically flexible. The cladding can be quite thin—on the order of tens of micrometers. The cladding is often protected by a jacket. This type of fiberguide is referred to as a step index, because of the abrupt change in refractive index between core and cladding. Another type of fiberguide is a gradient index (GRIN). The glass or other material is doped so that the refractive index varies with radius; it is maximum at the center. If a ray deviates from the axis, it is refracted back because of the gradient in the index.

Hundreds of fibers may be bundled together to transmit more light while maintaining flexibility. If no attempt is made to keep the fibers aligned, the bundle is called "incoherent" (not a good choice of terminology because of the possibility of confusing it with the coherence of a laser beam). There is additional loss because of the dead space between cylindrical fibers. If the fibers at the exit are in the same spatial relationship to one another as at the entrance, the bundle is called "coherent" and is an imageguide.

Imageguide

An image focused at the entrance end of an imageguide is dissected into thousands of elements, one fiber per element, and the light is transmitted to form an image at the exit end. For example, medical endoscopes are small and flexible enough to be guided through the respiratory tract, through the gastrointestinal tract, into joints, etc. An imageguide might be 1 mm by 1 mm, made up of fibers 10 μm in diameter, providing 10,000 picture elements (pixels). This is adequate for most applications. An example of an endoscope is shown in Fig. 5.13. The imageguide is used to guide the endoscope by eye (with the ocular at one end) or video camera, with the aid of wires built into the body of the scope. At least one open channel about 1 mm in diameter is provided for suctioning off fluids, collecting a biopsy specimen, performing surgery, etc. The use of endoscopes for surgery (including laser surgery) and diagnosis is a great advance.

5.4 DETECTORS AND ELECTRONICS

There are two types of optical detectors: thermal and photon. Thermal detectors are most appropriate for milliwatts to watts of power; they are too insensitive for low power. On the other hand, photon detectors may be damaged at high power and are most appropriate for low power (microwatts to milliwatts).

Thermal detectors convert light energy into heat energy by absorption in a blackened coating. The resulting increase in temperature is measured by a thermocouple or array of thermocouples (thermopile), by the change in resistance with temperature, or by a change in piezoelectric response. The ab-

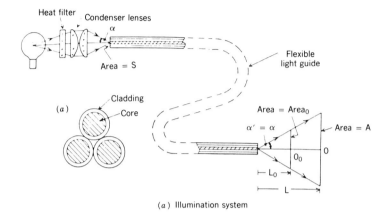

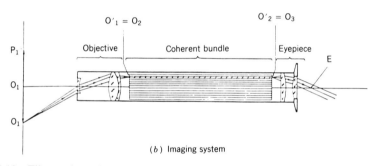

(b) Imaging system

FIG. 5.13   Fiberoptic endoscope, showing illumination and imaging systems. (Hopkins, H. H. 1972. In G. Berci (Ed.), *Endoscopy*. New York: Appleton-Century-Crofts.)

sorbant coating may be black over a wide range of wavelengths, hence thermal detectors typically have a flat response from the UV range to at least 10 µm, depending on the transmittance of the window. In photon detectors, the charge is released by absorption of photons in the detection medium without conversion to heat (photoelectric effect). It may be possible to detect single photons or, more commonly, to measure the average current by collecting the charge. The response of photon detectors is wavelength dependent, and there is a long wavelength limit corresponding to the minimum quantum energy required to release the charge (photoelectron, or hole-electron pair in a semiconductor). In addition to the wavelength dependence, selection of a detector requires consideration of the speed of response to a step change in incident power (or an equivalent frequency response for a modulated source), gain, output signal, output impedance, the maximum power with the required linearity, and the minimum detectable power (limited by detector noise).

Noise

Noise is very important in detecting weak radiation. Noise is frequency dependent, as discussed in Chapter 3. For example, at low frequencies the noise power often varies as $1/f$, and the noise voltage as $f^{-0.5}$. In the midrange of frequencies, semiconductor detector noise comes from generation and recombination of charge carriers and is independent of frequency. At high frequencies, the major source of noise is Johnson noise in the load resistor, and is independent of frequency ("white noise"). The magnitude of noise may be expressed as the noise equivalent power (NEP or P_N). This is defined as the input radiant power that produces an output with a signal to-noise-ratio of unity, for a specified electrical bandwidth Δf, often 1 Hz, as defined in equation 3.30.

Another way to look at it is that P_N is the smallest radiant power that can be measured when the signal integration time is about 1 second. A smaller P_N corresponds to better performance.

A useful "figure of merit" (larger for better signal-to-noise performance) is the specific detectivity. For a detector in which the noise is proportional to the square root of detector area A and the square root of the bandwidth, it is defined in equation 3.31.

Thermal Detectors

The thermal detectors include the bolometer, the thermopile, and the pyroelectric detector.

The **bolometer** element is a metal or thermistor, which changes resistance with temperature. A matched element, shielded from the incident optical radiation, is incorporated to compensate for variations in ambient temperature. Time constant is on the order of 1 to 15 ms, and it is advantageous to modulate or chop the source beam at 10 Hz and use a lock-in amplifier to optimize the signal-to-noise ratio. Specific detectivity may be about 2×10^8 cm $(Hz)^{-0.5}$ W^{-1}, less than that for some photon detectors.

The **thermopile** is a stack of interconnected thermocouples. The heat sink for the cold junction is located outside of the radiation beam. In one version, 64 couples of antimony and bismuth are vacuum deposited on a thin aluminum oxide window, backed by a gold-black absorber (gold evaporated in a poor vacuum so that the surface is rough and appears black or totally absorbing). Specific detectivity may be about 10^9 cm $Hz^{-0.5}$ W^{-1}. The time constant of a thermopile for response to a step increase in incident power may be 10 μs to 10 ms.

Pyroelectric Detector. Certain crystals, e.g., triglycene sulfate, lithium tantalate, strontium barium niobate, and polyvinylidene fluoride, are ferroelectric; that is, they are charged even in the absence of an applied electric field. Furthermore, the charge is very dependent on temperature. If gold electrodes, each of area A, are vacuum evaporated on two opposite faces and connected to an external load resistor or amplifier, a current flows,

$$i = pA \frac{dT}{dt}, \tag{5.16}$$

where p is the *pyroelectric* coefficient. As indicated by the expression, there is no current unless the temperature changes, hence there is no DC response and the radiation beam has to be chopped unless the light source itself is pulsed or otherwise modulated. The pyroelectric detector has an equivalent shunt resistance and capacitance, so the responsivity varies with frequency but can be up to 10 to 100 MHz, much faster than other thermal detectors. There is a range of frequencies in which responsivity is independent of frequency, but it does depend on the load resistance. For $R_L = 10^8 \Omega$, P_N for 1 Hz, bandwidth may be 10^{-8} W.

Photon Detectors

Photon detectors for optical radiation include photoemissive vacuum devices (photomultiplier tube or vacuum photodiode) and photoconductive or photovoltaic semiconductor diodes (photodiodes). The responsivity depends on wavelength, the material of the photocathode and window (photoemissive tube) or on the type of semiconductor.

The **photoemissive detector** consists of a special photocathode with low work function, an anode, and an electron multiplier (in a photomultiplier tube [PMT]). A schematic diagram of a PMT is shown in Fig. 5.14. When a photon impinges on the photocathode, it may transfer energy and eject a photoelectron with initial kinetic energy:

$$K = h\nu - \phi, \tag{5.17}$$

where $h\nu$ is the photon energy (Planck's constant times the frequency) and ϕ is the work function. Photons with energy less than ϕ cannot eject electrons, and this corresponds to the lowest frequency or longest wavelength that can be detected. The dynodes and, finally, the anode are supplied with a bias potential through the voltage divider, so that each is more positive than the photocathode, or preceding dynode, by about 75 or 100 V. The dynode surfaces are coated or treated so that emission of secondary electrons is facilitated (e.g., Cs_3Sb, Cu-BeO-Cs, GaP:Cs). Thus, there is a multiplication of charge as the photoelectron is accelerated and focused to hit the first dynode, the secondary electrons emitted are accelerated and focused on the second dynode, etc., until finally the multipled electrons are collected at the anode. The gain is expressed as

$$G = \delta^n, \tag{5.18}$$

where δ is the number of secondary electrons per incident electron (a function of the accelerating voltage and dynode material), and n is the number of

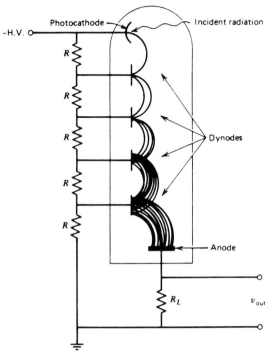

FIG. 5.14 Schematic of photomultiplier tube. (Boyd, R. W. 1983. *Radiometry and the detection of optical radiation*. New York: John Wiley & Sons.)

dynodes. In a typical photomultiplier tube, $\delta = 4$, $n = 9$, and $G = 3 \times 10^5$. Similar gains can be achieved with a microchannel plate-type multiplier.

Photocathodes may be opaque (side window tube), or thin and semitransparent (end window tube), so that the photoelectrons can escape. Figure 5.15 plots the responsivity (in mA per watt of radiant power) as a function of wavelength for some photocathode materials and windows. (The transmission of light through the window limits the response, especially at short wavelengths.) The Ag-O-Cs photocathode is often designated as the S-1 response. The Cs_3Sb photocathode has various S designations, depending on details of processing and window material (S-11 is shown in the figure). The $Na_2KSb:Cs$ photocathode is called multialkali or S-20. ERMA-II and ERMA-III are extended red multialkali photocathodes with increased red response, achieved mostly by using a thicker cathode. The GaAs:Cs-O photocathode is termed a negative electron affinity material. (For an explanation, see Boyd, listed in the Bibliography at the end of this chapter.)

The speed of response of photoemissive detectors is very good, 10^{-8} to 10^{-9} seconds. Noise arises mainly from thermal electrons emitted from the photocathode (although there is a small contribution from the statistical nature of electron multiplication) and can be reduced by cooling. The dark current

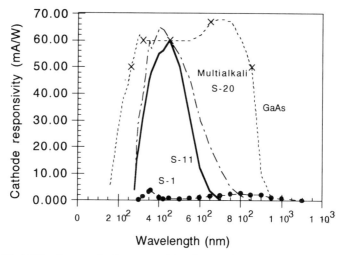

FIG. 5.15 Photocathode responsivity (mA/W) vs. wavelength (nm).

leaving the photocathode is approximated by

$$i_D = 120\,AT^2\,\exp\frac{-\phi}{kT}, \tag{5.19}$$

where the cathode area A is expressed in cm² and T in degrees Kelvin. For a photocathode in which $\phi = 1.24$ eV (cutoff wavelength 1 μm), at 300 K, 1 cm² of photocathode will emit a dark current of about 2×10^{-14} A. Assuming $\Delta f = 1$ Hz and 10 percent quantum efficiency, $P_N = 10^{-14}$ W (see Boyd, listed in this chapter's Bibliography). The dark current will be multiplied by the same gain factor as the signal current.

Photodiodes are operated as reverse-biased junction diodes with a bias potential of about 15 V and with a surface exposed to the light. Detection of optical radiation with a photodiode is based on measuring the variation with the illumination of either the voltage generated (photovoltaic diode [PV]) or the current through a semiconductor whose resistance varies with the illumination (photoconductive diode [PC]). The specific detectivity of an infrared-sensitive PV detector is somewhat better than for an equivalent PC detector, but the speed of response is not as good. Absorption of light imparts energy to a valence electron, elevating it to the conduction band. A hole, which acts as a positive charge, is left. Both electrons and holes migrate in the applied electric field, constituting the current. A contact difference of potential exists even when no external voltage is applied, corresponding to that of a photovoltaic detector. The measuring circuits are shown in Fig. 5.16. The responsivity as a function of wavelength for some representative semiconductors is given in Fig. 5.17. The minimum photon energy that can be detected corresponds to the bandgap energy of the semiconductor. Noise is

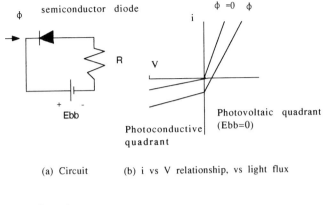

(a) Circuit   (b) i vs V relationship, vs light flux

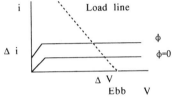

(c) Change in i or V with light flux on photoconductive diode

FIG. 5.16 Circuits and characteristics of reverse-biased photoconductive and photovoltaic semiconductor diode light sensors.

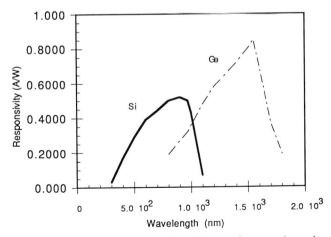

FIG. 5.17 Responsivity vs. wavelength for silicon and germanium photodiodes.

reduced and specific detectivity increased by operation at low temperatures, e.g., 77 K (boiling point of liquid nitrogen at atmospheric pressure). Response times may vary from 0.1 to 30 ms.

For detection of visible light and longer wavelength UV, the room-temperature silicon detector is quite suitable, although the detectivity of PC and PV detectors is only about 1 percent of that for a PMT. Speed of response is on the order of microseconds.

Camera

The PMT and photodiode are used in most biomedical engineering applications where imaging is not required. Imaging is performed by a video camera or by a camera and image intensifier. The standard camera now uses a charge-coupled device (CCD). The photodetector consists of thousands of silicon photodiodes (one for each pixel in a video frame), which detect and integrate light until the charge is read out during the video frame (1/30 second). The frame diagonal is typically 18 mm or 13 mm, and the aspect ratio (vertical dimension by horizontal dimension) is 3:4 in the U.S. standard. Packets of charge are moved sequentially to a register by high-frequency clock pulses. Some noise occurs from thermally released electrons; it is minimized by cooling the CCD array with a Peltier device. The CCD camera is suitable for illumination from daylight to 5 lux.

Image Intensifier

Imaging may be performed at low light levels using an image intensifier. The modern high-vacuum image intensifier amplifies the image brightness light by conversion into a pattern of charge in a photocathode, charge multiplication in a microchannel plate (MCP), and excitation of phosphorescence by the electrons striking a semitransparent phosphor deposit. The phosphor emission is usually green for viewing by eye. The responsivity of the photocathode depends on the material, as with PMTs.

A cross section of the Gen II or Gen III image intensifier is given in Fig. 5.18. Such a device is often called a *proximity focus tube*, because there is no electrostatic or magnetic focusing, only the small gaps between the pho-

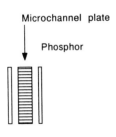

Microchannel plate

Phosphor

Photocathode

FIG. 5.18 Proximity focus image intensifier. The microchannel plate amplifies the electron current by secondary electron emission.

tocathode, MCP, and anode of the phosphor to keep the electrons from an image point from spreading. The MCP contains thousands of closely spaced, etched longitudinal holes, each a few micrometers in diameter, coated with a semiconducting layer. A voltage across the MCP accelerates the electrons, and the electrons are multilied by secondary emission. There is also a voltage applied between the photocathode and the MCP, and between the MCP and the phosphor-coated anode. The relationship between screen luminance and photocathode illuminance is linear, unless automatic gain control is provided for the MCP gain by varying its voltage.

5.5 RADIOMETRY AND PHOTOMETRY

Optical sensors or detectors measure radiant power (flux) in the optical region of the electromagnetic spectrum (UV, visible, infrared). Other radiometric measurands (exitance, irradiance, intensity, radiance, energy fluence rate), can be derived from the power as measured in certain geometries. If the detector is made to respond like the light-adapted eye, one can define the equivalent of power, the lumen. The corresponding photometric quantities can then be derived (luminous exitance, illuminance, luminous intensity, and luminance).

Radiometry

Radiometry refers to the measurement or calculation of the flow of light power or energy. If the spectrum is also measured or calculated, it may be considered as spectroradiometry. The fundamental quantity in radiometry is power (watts) or, if integrated over time, energy (joules). Historically, associated quantities have been defined with regard to an opaque surface, either in terms of power received or emitted per unit area of the surface (W/m^2 or W/cm^2), or as the power per unit area and per unit solid angle (W/m^2 sr or W/cm^2 sr), where sr is steradian. (This applies as well to the flux emerging from a surface.) Also of interest is the power per unit area oriented perpendicular to the light ray, or entering a sphere of unit cross-sectional area, as this quantity times a cross section gives a reaction rate. This quantity is now called the *radiant energy fluence rate*, (formerly termed the *space irradiance*). The symbol F is used for this quantity. Intensity refers to the power per unit solid angle. Radiometric quantities are summarized in Table 5.3.

Photometry

If the spectrum is weighted by the response of the scotopic (light-adapted) eye, the corresponding photometric quantities are obtained. The weighting function V_λ is plotted in Fig. 5.19. Radiant flux is replaced by luminous flux,

TABLE 5.3   Radiometric Quantities

Radiant flux	ϕ (W)	Power carried by beam
Radiance	L (W m^{-2} sr)	Power per unit area and solid angle
Irradiance	E (W m^{-2})	Power incident on 1 m^2 surface area
Exitance	M (W m^{-2})	Power emitted by 1 m^2 surface area
Fluence rate	F (W m^{-2})	Power entering 1 m^2 cross section sphere
(Space irradiance)		
Intensity	I (W sr^{-1})	Power per unit solid angle

Note: If spectral quantities are involved, ϕ is replaced by $\phi(\lambda)$ (W nm^{-1}). If photometric quantities are involved, ϕ is replaced by ϕ_v and W is replaced by lumen.

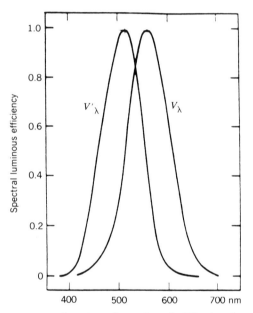

FIG. 5.19   Eye response as a function of wavelength. *V* is the photometric weighting function with 1 watt = 680 lumens at 555 nm. *V'* is for the dark-adapted eye, in relative units. (Boyd, R. W. 1983. *Radiometry and the detection of optical radiation.* New York: John Wiley & Sons.)

the unit being a lumen instead of a watt. The relationship is expressed as follows:

$$680 \text{ lumens} = 1 \text{ W, at } \lambda = 555 \text{ nm (maximum response)}. \quad (5.20)$$

Then radiance becomes luminance, irradiance becomes illuminance, radiant exitance becomes luminous exitance, the equivalent of radiant energy fluence rate or space irradiance becomes a luminous quantity, and radiant intensity becomes luminous intensity. Instruments are often described in terms of luminous quantities at a specified "color temperature," describing an equivalent blackbody at that temperature (e.g., 3000 K). Radiometric quantities are useful when the eye response is not involved, and apply even outside the visible spectrum.

Measurement of Radiometric Quantities

Typical geometries for measuring radiometric quantities are illustrated in Fig. 5.20. Flux (power) is measured with a photoelectric detector of known responsitivity (e.g., V/W). The responsivity may be calculated from the basic interactions and charge collection efficiency, or calibrated against a standard lamp. A standard lamp is typically a quartz-halogen tungsten incandescent bulb with a precisely made filament, powered by a precision constant-current

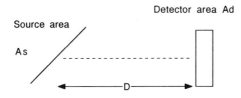

(a) Irradiance or flux

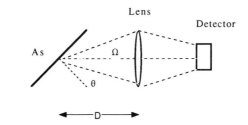

(b) radiance, lens subtends solid angle Ω

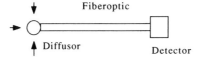

(c) Energy fluence rate

FIG. 5.20 Geometries for measurement of radiometric quantities: **(a)** measurement of irradiance or flux, **(b)** measurement of radiance, **(c)** measurement of energy fluence rate (space irradiance).

power supply. In the infrared range, a blackbody may used in which a beam is extracted from a small hole in a large electrically heated cavity, held at constant temperature. The output radiance of the standard lamp is known, as well as the spectrum. If the sensitivity of the photodetector is independent of wavelength (over some defined band), the total flux can be measured. If the sensitivity is wavelength dependent, the response has to be weighted by the spectrum, or the power measured per unit wavelength using a grating monochromator or a series of narrow bandpass filters. The calibrated detector responds only to the light incident; thus, if a collimated beam is to be measured, its diameter should be less than the dimensions of the detector. The detector is usually perpendicular to the beam.

The irradiance is determined by measuring the flux and dividing by the sensitive area of the detector, provided the incident light overfills the detector aperture. If the beam is smaller, the irradiated area should be used instead.

Radiance measurements involve both an area and a solid angle. If the radiance of light emitted by a large area source is of concern, the detector is fitted with a lens that defines the solid angle, assuming the detector aperture is overfilled. In general,

$$L = \frac{E}{\Omega'} = \frac{ED^2}{A_s \cos \theta} = \frac{vD^2}{R_E A_s \cos \theta} \ (\text{W cm}^{-2} \ \text{sr}^{-1}), \qquad (5.21)$$

where L is the source radiance, E the measured irradiance at the detector entrance aperture, Ω' the solid angle subtended by the source at the detector entrance aperture (e.g., as defined by a collimator or a lens of typically either $3°$ or $8°$ acceptance angle), D the distance from the source to the entrance aperture, A_s the source area, θ the angle between the source normal and the optical axis of the radiometer, R_E the responsivity of the detector to irradiance, and v the measured signal (volts).

Energy fluence rate (space irradiance) is the radiance integrated over 4π solid angle. It can be measured with an isotropic detector. For example, the tip of a fiberoptic lightguide can be coated with a light-diffusing material that will scatter light into the lightguide equally, regardless of the angle of incidence (within limits; response is lower where shaded by the fiber itself). The opposite end of the lightguide is coupled to the photodetector. The device is calibrated by reading the response (volts) in a transparent medium with the diffusing tip irradiated by a collimated beam. The irradiance of the beam can be measured; in beam geometry the energy fluence rate is equal to the irradiance. An experimental correction has to be applied if the refractive index of the transparent medium is different from the refractive index of the medium in which the actual measurement of energy fluence rate is to be made. The reason is that the scattering into and out of the diffusing material depends on the refractive indexes of diffuser and medium.

5.6   TISSUE OPTICS

Tissue optics is concerned with the propagation of light in and through tissue. An issue of the journal *Applied Optics*, including papers based on a symposium, is devoted to tissue optics (see this chapter's Bibliography).

Tissue is a turbid medium, in which light is scattered and absorbed. For a steady source, the radiance at a given position obeys the Boltzmann transport equation:

$$\nabla \cdot L(\Omega) + \mu_t L(\Omega) = \int \mu_s S(\theta) L(\Omega')d\Omega' + Q(\Omega'), \qquad (5.22)$$

where $L(\Omega)$ is the radiance after scattering, $L(\Omega')$ is the radiance before scattering through angle θ, $S(\theta)$ is the normalized angular distribution of scattering (phase function), μ_t is the total interaction coefficient (absorption plus scattering, $\mu_a + \mu_s$), and Q is the source density.

The Boltzmann transport equation is solved subject to boundary conditions, e.g., no return of photons to the exterior surface. Boundary conditions are also applied for surface sources. If the refractive indexes within and outside the boundary are not matched, some of the energy is reflected according to the Fresnel relationship:

$$\{(1 - p)/(1 + p)\}^2, \qquad (5.23)$$

where $p = n_1/n_2$ th ratio of the refractive index before the boundary and after the boundary, and only a fraction of the energy enters the turbid medium.

The radiant energy fluence rate is the integral of the radiance over 4π solid angle:

$$F = \int_{4\pi} L(\Omega) \, d\Omega. \qquad (5.24)$$

Equation 5.22 can be solved by the discrete ordinates method or the Monte Carlo method.

Discrete Ordinates

In the discrete ordinates method, equation 5.24 is written as a finite integro-difference equation (subject to boundary conditions), with energy in energy intervals (groups), position as cells with an average and certain edge coordinates, and angle as magnitudes at given angles (as cosines μ_m) and weights, w_m. A distinguishing characteristic of the discrete ordinates method is the representation of direction in the fixed laboratory coordinate system in terms of a few angles. The (μ_m, w_m) system is analogous to a quadrature scheme for integration. The equation is solved by iteration, starting with an arbitrary guess. The relationship between one cell and the next may be written in terms of the diamond difference model or the finite difference model. (See *Radiation Shielding and Dosimetry*, by Profio, listed in this chapter's Bibliography, for this detail and other information on the discrete ordinates method, pages 199–218.) The discrete ordinates method is especially suited for one-dimensional geometries (sphere, infinite cylinder, infinite planar slab). Two-dimensional and time-dependent calculations can also be performed, but the computer memory size and computation time increase rapidly with increasing dimensionality.

Monte Carlo

The Monte Carlo method is essentially a computer simulation of an experiment, as diagrammed in Fig. 5.21. A number of special-purpose Monte Carlo programs have been developed for computation of the transport of light. One advantage with this method for light transport is that there is no change of energy, hence wavelength, in scattering. The Monte Carlo method can be used for three-dimensional and time-dependent problems.

The essence of the method is selection of a variable from a cumulative distribution function (CDF) with the aid of a random number (r) between 0 and 1. The CDF is the sum of the partial distribution functions (PDFs).

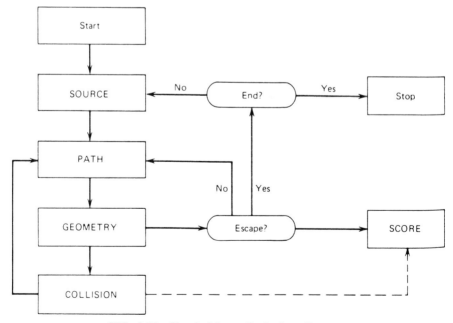

FIG. 5.21 Simple Monte Carlo flow diagram.

The CDF is set equal to r, from which the PDFs are derived, as shown in Fig. 5.22, for selection between scattering and absorption. In this example, PDF μ_a/μ_t for absorption is 0.4, whereas the PDF μ_s/μ_t for scattering is 0.6. If a random number between 0.0 and 0.4 is selected, then the photon is assumed to be absorbed. If r is between 0.4 and 1.0, then scattering is assumed to occur in the computer simulation. Note that r is actually a computed pseudorandom number.

The source routine sets the initial energy, position (x, y, z), and direction (angle). The direction is specified by direction cosines u, v, and w. The distance s to the next collision is distributed exponentially, hence,

$$s = -ln\ r. \tag{5.25}$$

The new position coordinates are computed from trigonometry.

A test is made to determine whether a boundary between media is crossed by comparing the coordinates with the coordinates of the boundaries specified by quartic surfaces (e.g., for an infinite cylinder of radius R, $x^2 + y^2 - R^2$). If an external boundary is crossed, the photon is assumed to escape and another photon is initiated by the source routine. If the photon remains in the same medium, the type of interaction (absorption or scattering) is selected through a CDF. The angle of scattering is chosen with another, continuous, CDF. The new direction is obtained from the old direction and the scattering angle with a transformation formula given in *Radiation Shielding and Dosimetry*, by Profio, page 186, listed in this chapter's Bibliography. The simulation then continues. Interactions are scored, e.g., when a boundary is crossed or an absorption occurs.

A problem with the Monte Carlo method is a relatively large statistical error, even when some 10,000 photons are started at the source, so that practical calculations use some method of variance reduction. More infor-

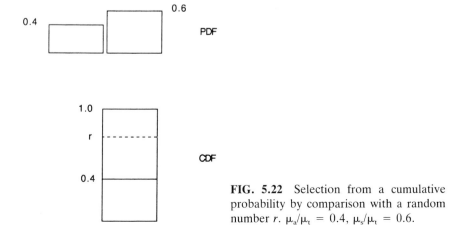

FIG. 5.22 Selection from a cumulative probability by comparison with a random number r. $\mu_a/\mu_t = 0.4$, $\mu_s/\mu_t = 0.6$.

mation may be found in Profio, *Radiation Shielding and Dosimetry*, pp. 168–199, listed in the Bibliography at the end of this chapter.

Interaction Coefficients

Absorption, scattering, and total interaction coefficients have to be measured. The phase function may be approximated by the Henyey-Greenstein function:

$$S(\theta) = \frac{(\mu_s/\mu_t)\ (1 - g^2)}{(1 + g^2 - 2g\ \cos\theta)^{3/2}}, \qquad (5.26)$$

and the average cosine of the scattering angle

$$g = \frac{\int_{4\pi} S(\theta)\ \cos\theta\ d\Omega}{\int_{4\pi} S(\theta)\ d\Omega}. \qquad (5.27)$$

It is also possible to measure $S(\theta)$.

The total interaction coefficient at a given wavelength is measured with the tissue specimen in a very well collimated beam from the source to detector. It is advisable to monitor the source power as well, for example, by using a beamsplitter and photodiode. A suitable apparatus is depicted in Fig. 5.23. The absorption coefficient can be derived from the absorbance relative to a standard in an integrating sphere (a sphere with a diffusing coating). The scattering coefficient is the difference between the total and absorption coefficients. The phase function is measured with a goniometer.

Diffusion Theory

If absorption is small, as compared with scattering, and the position is far from a boundary or localized source, then diffusion theory often gives a satisfactory approximation of the energy fluence rate (F). Diffusion theory is most useful in one-dimensional geometry (for a homogeneous sphere or nested spherical shells with an isotropic point source at the center; infinitely long cylinder or cylindrical shells with an isotropic line source along the axis; infinitely broad slab or laminated slabs with a planar source on one side, usually approximated by a perpendicularly incident collimated beam). If the slab material is not matched in refractive index with the material containing the source, an experimental or computational correction should be applied. The diffusion equation is

$$D\ \nabla^2 F - \mu_a F + Q = 0, \qquad (5.28)$$

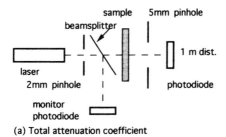

(a) Total attenuation coefficient

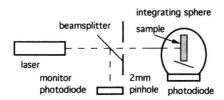

(b) Absorbance apparatus: compare sample absorbance to diffuser

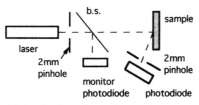

(c) Angular dependence of scattering

FIG. 5.23 Experimental arrangements for measuring optical properties of samples. (Adapted from Marchesini, R., A. Bertoni, S. Andreola, et al., Extinction and absorption coefficients and scattering phase functions of human tissue in vitro," 1984. *Appl. Optics* 28:2319–2320.)

where the diffusion coefficient

$$D = \frac{1}{3[\mu_a + \mu_s(1 - g)]} \tag{5.29}$$

and the (diffuse) attenuation coefficient or inverse of the diffusion length

$$\alpha = \sqrt{\frac{\mu_a}{D}}. \tag{5.30}$$

A better approximation of radiation transport, for values close to $1/\alpha$ from a pencil beam or similar source, is to add the solution of equation 5.28 to the solution for a collimated beam. For example, for a beam along the $+x$ axis is planar geometry,

$$F_x = F_{xo} \ (\exp \ -\mu_t x), \tag{5.31}$$

and this expression may be used for the volume source.

Diffusion Parameters

The *attenuation coefficient* can be obtained by measuring F versus x in planar geometry, for x large compared with $1/\mu_t$, where x is the distance from the source plane:

$$F(x) = F_o \exp (-\alpha x) \tag{5.32}$$

and F_o is the energy fluence rate at the source.

The *diffusion coefficient* (D) may be measured by the "poisoned moderator" technique, in which α is measured as a function of added absorption $\delta\mu_a$. Then, by plotting α^2 vs $\delta\mu_a$ and using equation 5.30, a line is obtained whose slope is $1/D$ and whose zero intercept μ_a corresponds to the absorption by the original medium (e.g., tissue).

A typical value for μ_t is 320 to 700 cm^{-1} at 630 nm, and in a lightly absorbing medium, μ_s is about the same, assuming near isotropic scattering. The value of μ_a is about 1 cm^{-1} in typical tissue, and g is 0.64 to 0.97, all at 630 nm.

One can also simply measure F(x). Figure 5.24 compares results for an expanded helium-neon laser beam in a phantom suspension of Evans blue absorber in Intralipid (fat globules) scatterer. Table 5.4 lists measured values of the optical diffusion length (δ) in specimens of various tissues, and at selected laser wavelengths.

5.7 LASER SURGERY

Laser-tissue interactions are plotted in Fig. 5.25 as a function of radiant exposure (irradiance integrated over time) and exposure duration, for a pulsed source. Pulsing is introduced because the conduction of heat takes some time. The dividing lines between different interactions are approximate. Some temperatures and lasers are also indicated in Fig. 5.25. Multiphoton and some less common effects have been omitted.

Lasers are used in medicine for incision and for explosive ablation of tumors and other tissues, for blood vessel coagulation in various tissues, including the retina and port-wine stain birthmarks, and for photo disruption of the lens capsule. Most effects can be explained by heating or optical breakdown (photochemical effects are discussed in Section 5.8). Coagulation occurs as the temperature is increased, then ablation and, finally, carbonization. The

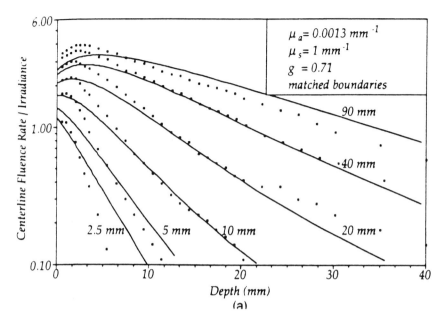

FIG. 5.24 Comparison of measured (*dotted curve*) vs. diffusion theory calculation (*solid curve*) for perpendicularly incident beam of 2.5 mm to 90 mm diameter, on slab phantom, with refractive index matched at boundaries. (From Moes, C. J. M., M. J. C. van Gemert, Willem M. Star, et al. 1989. Measurement of the energy fluence rate in a scattering and absorbing phantom at 633 nm. *Applied Optics* 28[12].)

TABLE 5.4   Optical Penetration Depth δ (mm) at Various Wavelengths

	Wavelength (nm)			
Tissue	488/515	630	660/665	1064
Brain, white matter	0.4–1.7		1.2–5.4	3.2–8.8
Astrocytoma	0.5–1.3		2.0–3.0	3.0–6.3
Glioblastoma multiforme	1.4		6.6	
Bladder wall		1.9		
Bladder carcinoma		2.2–2.3		
Bronchial mucosa		1.1		
Lung, deflated		0.9		
Bronchial carcinoma		1.6		
Aortic wall, partially calcified	0.2–0.4	0.7–1.0		
Aortic wall, necrosis		0.4		
Adipose	0.7	1.8		
Retinoblastoma, mouse	1.6	3.3	3.6	7.5

Note: At 10.6 μm, δ = 0.03 mm for most tissues because of absorption in water. Courtesy of L.O. Svaasand, Univ. of Trondheim, Norway.

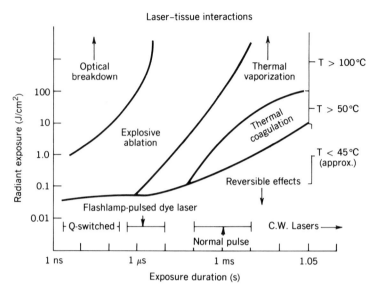

FIG. 5.25   Laser-tissue interactions vs. radiant exposure and pulse duration. (From Sliney, D. H. 1989. *Dosimetry of laser radiation in medicine and biology*. Vol. IS-5, p. 7, Bellingham, Wash: SPIE.)

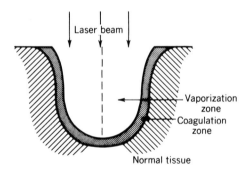

FIG. 5.26   Laser cut.

cut from a laser is shown in Fig. 5.26. Ablation can be analyzed in terms of strongly pulsed superheating of the tissue. Thus it is important to consider the temperature-time-position dependence as a function of pulse duration (and repetition rate at high rates) as well as irradiance or exposure.

Steady-state heat transfer is discussed in Chapter 4, Section 4.7 (Thermal Models). The thermal source density is given by

$$q = \mu_a F. \tag{5.33}$$

Calculation

Assume the tissue is heated by absorption of light. F, the energy fluence rate, is derived as discussed in Section 5.6 (Tissue Optics).

In laser surgery the laser is often pulsed in order to limit the volume heated to a high temperature. If the pulse width is small as compared with the blood perfusion transport time, cooling by blood is unimportant at short times and the process is controlled by thermal conduction. The dynamic thermal behavior is characterized by the ratio between the thermal conductivity and specific heat per unit volume, which is known as the thermal diffusivity:

$$\chi = \frac{\kappa}{\rho C}. \tag{5.34}$$

The thermal diffusivity of most tissues is 1.2×10^{-7} m^2/s^4.

Cooling from blood perfusion is insignificant as compared with thermal conduction if the light is absorbed in a linear dimension that is small as compared with the thermal penetration depth. Then T can be calculated from the time-dependent heat transfer equation (with blood transport neglected). An example of the temperature (in arbitrary units) as a function of depth at various times after absorption of a short pulse of radiation absorbed at the surface of a plane slab (e.g., from a CO_2 laser) is shown in Fig. 5.27, compared to measurements (dots). Approximately, the time τ required for heat to diffuse to a depth d is

$$\tau = d^2/\chi. \tag{5.35}$$

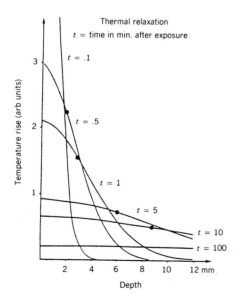

FIG. 5.27   Temperature (arbitrary units) vs. distance from pulsed heat source in tissue, thermal diffusivity $\chi = 1.2 \times 10^{-7}$ m^2/s at various times (minutes). (From Svaasand, L. O., C. J. Gomer, A. J. Welch, 1989. Thermotics of tissue. In *Dosimetry of laser radiation in medicine and biology*. Vol. IS5, p. 135. Edited by G. J. Miller and D. H. Sliney. Bellingham, Wash: SPIE Optical Engineering Press.)

For a rough approximation when thermal conduction can be neglected (e.g., during and immediately after an intense short laser pulse), the energy deposited by the laser in a critical volume raises the temperature to the coagulation or vaporization point. The critical volume is defined as having the area (spot size) of the laser beam, A_s, and a thickness equal to the extinction length, $1/\alpha$, of the light of the laser wavelength in tissue. At the CO_2 laser wavelength, 10.6 µm, water is strongly absorbing, scattering is negligible, and $1/\alpha$ is 0.03 mm. When the absorbed energy in the critical volume $V_c = A_s/\alpha$ reaches 2500 J/cm^2, water is vaporized. The time required can be computed by knowing the beam power density, P/A_s (W/cm^2). A typical medical CO_2 laser is operated at 10 to 100 W for less than a second or so at a time, with $A_s = 0.01$ cm^2; hence a peak power density on the order of 10^3 to 10^4 W/cm^2. The laser is best suited for precise incision or tissue removal and can also serve for hemostasis of capillary vessels.

A Nd: YAG (or Nd:glass) laser operated at about 100 W is often used for tissue cutting and necrotization of a volume of tissue of 10 mm^3 or so. Larger blood vessels are coagulated (hemostasis). At the 1.06 µm wavelength, tissue is strongly scattering, absorption is relatively low, and the attenuation length $1/\alpha$ is about 2 to 3 mm. Considerable backscattering and optical diffusion occurs. Often the conduction of heat to surrounding tissue must be taken into account, so the approximation of no heat loss is inaccurate. Because of the thermal as well as optical diffusion, the damaged volume is typically a few millimeters in diameter and a few millimeters in depth.

Measurement

Temperature is usually measured with a Chromel-Alumel thermocouple a few tenths of a millimeter in diameter, including insulation and jacket. Often the thermocouple is built into a hypodermic needle, which is inserted into the tissue.

5.8   PHOTODYNAMIC THERAPY

Phototherapy is the treatment of disease by exposure to light, at such powers and power densities that heating is of little or no importance as compared with the effects of photochemistry. A particular form, photodynamic therapy (PDT), has undergone much development in recent years for treatment of malignant tumors, and, lately, for removal of atherosclerotic deposits.

In PDT, a drug is injected that preferentially accumulates in the target tissue, e.g., a tumor, while it is substantially cleared after some time from normal surrounding tissues. The reason for the selectivity is not clear. The drug used most often has been termed *hematoporphyrin-derivative* (HpD) or *dihematoporphyrin ether/ester* (DHE). The drug is now available commercially and approved for human use. Upon exposure to light, in the presence of ordinary molecular oxygen, not only is the drug excited, but also molecular oxygen is excited to a higher energy state (which happens to be singlet), and the product is "singlet oxygen."

Photochemistry and Physics

The absorption of light by the photosensitizer ^1S initially converts it to the excited singlet state, $^1S^*$:

$$^1S + hv \rightarrow 1S^*.$$

Some of the absorbed energy is radiated as fluorescence (with a broad spectrum in the red, and a lifetime on the order of a few nanoseconds). Nonradiative processes (physical and chemical quenching or heating) may occur. The excited sensitizer may transfer energy by a process termed *intersystem crossover*:

$$^1S^* \rightarrow {}^3S.$$

The triplet-state sensitizer can then transfer energy to oxygen and excite it to singlet oxygen:

$$^3S + {}^3O_2 \rightarrow {}^1O_2$$

The singlet oyxgen oxidizes biomolecules and leads to the tissue effects.

The radiative deexcitation of singlet oxygen results in infrared phosphorescence (1270 nm; lifetime depends on solvent and other effects, but is on the order of microseconds). Oxidation of biomolecules may be considered as chemical quenching, and physical quenching may also occur.

Properties of DHE: Skin Photosensitivity

The absorption coefficient of DHE is plotted against wavelength in Fig. 5.28. The wavelength used in clinical situations is 630 nm from an argon-dye laser (or 628 nm from a gold-vapor laser), corresponding to an absorption peak. Although the absorption is larger at wavelengths less than some 600 nm, the transport of light in tissue is less because of the absorption by hemoglobin and other constituents of tissue, and scattering; therefore, 630 nm is preferred for treatment of thick tumors (on the order of 1 cm).

The drug dosage has been determined empirically that will provide a concentration in the tumor suitable for PDT with a power density of less than 100 mW/cm^2 (so that heating is negligible). A dosage of about 2.0 mg DHE per kilogram of body weight in the human adult is standard and results in a concentration on the order of 1 to 10 µg/g of tissue in malignant tumors.

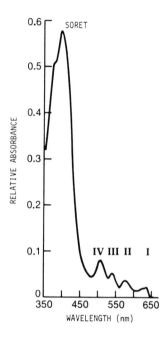

FIG. 5.28 Absorption of DHE vs. wavelength.

Lower dosages and concentrations may be adequate. The concentration stays high in a malignant tumor for days to months, whereas the concentration in nonmalignant tissues decreases over a few days. A delay of 24 to 72 hours is sufficient for clearance of most of the DHE from normal tissues. However, some DHE remains in the skin for a few weeks, leading to the major side effect of PDT: sensitivity to sunlight or other bright light. The effect may be slight erythema to blistering of the skin, but is entirely controllable by covering the skin with clothing or a visible-lightblocking sunscreen lotion.

Light Irradiation

A good deal of engineering has gone into design for the irradiation of tissue. The basic principles of the radiant energy fluence calculations and measurements are discussed in Section 5.6, Tissue Optics. Common irradiation geometries include (1) irradiation from an expanded laser beam or fiberoptic lightguide, such that the spot is considerably larger than the diameter of the tumor, usually with near perpendicular incidence, (2) irradiation from a diffusing fiberoptic lightguide inserted into the lumen of a body tube or cavity, and (3) a diffusing tip, isotropic lightguide or multiple lightguides, inserted interstitially into the tumor. The diffusion of light is assisted by stripping the cladding from the end of the fiber and coating the core with a scatterer such as aluminum oxide in synthetic resin. The length and composition of the coating is adjusted to maintain as uniform an irradiation as possible over the tumor.

The radiant energy fluence rate (F) will vary with distance from the irradiator in any case. If the concentration of DHE in the tumor is only 10 times as great as in surrounding tissue (an estimate), then F_{min} at the least irradiated point in the tumor should not be less than $0.1F_{max}$, assuming the most irradiated point is F_{max}. The attenuation length, $1/\alpha$, is typically about 0.3 to 0.4 cm in most tissues, at 630 nm. Thus, with exponential attenuation, $3 \propto (0.9–1.2 cm)$ gives $F_{min} = 0.05F_{max}$. It is standard practice to design the irradiation so that the thickest tumor treated is less than 1 cm, or to use multiple fibers spaced about 1 cm apart.

Empirically, in planar geometry, an irradiance (E) of about 100 J/cm^2 is sufficient for eradication of tumors. F at the surface may be up to 4E because of backscattering, although 1.5E to 2.0E is more likely. The points in the tumor nearest the light source are overirradiated so that the least irradiated point receives adequate F to prevent regrowth.

Dosimetry

Dosimetry for PDT is still under investigation. The effective absorbed dose may be defined as

$$D_{eff} = (\mu/\rho) \ C \ F \ K, \tag{5.38}$$

where (μ/ρ) is the mass absorption coefficient of the photosensitizer, C is the concentration of photosensitizer, and K is a ratio of biological effects (or singlet oxygen production), which takes into account differences in oxygenation of the tissue. One approach is to measure the concentration of DHE by fluorescence or another method (such as reflectance), calculate or measure F, and perhaps measure the concentration of oxygen to determine K.

Another approach is to measure the production of singlet oxygen by specific chemical reactions or, perhaps, the infrared phosphorescence at 1270 nm, but this is difficult.

Biological Effects

Direct cell killing occurs in cell culture and may occur at sufficiently large doses in clinical practice. However, there is evidence that interruption of the blood supply to a tumor occurs at considerably lower doses, either through clotting of blood or breakdown of the endothelial cells of the capillaries. The photodynamic reaction depends on the presence of molecular oxygen; therefore it is possible that the photochemical effect may be decreased. On the other hand, the cells cannot survive without oxygen, so in practice the tumor becomes necrotic.

5.9 FLUORESCENCE DIAGNOSIS

The fluorescence of certain tumor-accumulating compounds, such as DHE, may be used for detection of even very small tumors. The fluorescence excitation spectrum is similar to the absorption spectrum, with a peak near 400 nm for DHE or its monomers. The violet excitation is preferred to locate a thin tumor at the surface, for example, in detection of bronchial carcinoma in situ. However, excitation at 630 nm or intermediate wavelengths may be chosen for thicker or underlying tumors. The exciting light is typically conducted from the laser to a possible tumor site through a fiberoptic lightguide. A single-filament, fused quartz fiberoptic lightguide is used for the violet excitation, inserted in the biopsy channel or the endoscope. At longer wavelengths, the fiberoptic lightguide already built into the endoscope for white-light illumination may be used for excitation.

The fluorescence emission spectrum of HpD/DHE is shown in Fig. 5.29. There are peaks at 630 nm and 690 nm. However, tissue is fluorescent even without injection of DHE, and this autofluorescence background is the main problem involved in fluorescence diagnosis with DHE. On the other hand, there are differences in the fluorescence spectrum of tumors as compared with normal tissue, and this may be exploited in future work.

Imaging Method

The fluorescence emission can be imaged by a red filter (e.g., at 690 nm) and an image intensifier (luminance gain about 40,000) coupled to an endoscope.

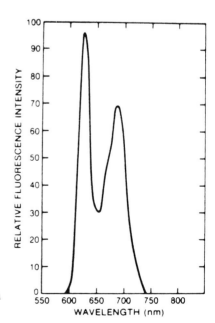

FIG. 5.29 Fluorescence emission spectrum of DHE.

The irradiance should be about 10 mW/cm², filling the field of view, with illumination as even as possible to avoid confusing a concentrated spot with an actual increase in the concentration of a fluorescent agent. If an endoscope is not needed, the image intensifier is probably not required either. The output of the image intensifier may be observed by eye or by a video camera.

The autofluorescence background may be subtracted by alternately imaging the autofluorescence with a green filter, for example, and the autofluorescence plus DHE fluorescence with a red filter. A scaled fraction of the green image is subtracted from the red image, assuming the shape of the autofluorescence spectrum is the same for nontumor and tumor sites so that the same scaling factor can be used. This is not necessarily true, but in practice background subtraction often helps in detection. A recent development is simultaneous red and green imaging, using two video cameras and a computer.

Guidance of the endoscope through the body, comparison with anatomical landmarks, and examination of suspicious sites is facilitated by switching on demand between the fluorescence image and a color reflectance image obtained under whitelight illumination.

Nonimaging Method

In the nonimaging method, simultaneous measurements of green- and red-filtered fluorescence emission are made on light conducted by a fiberoptic lightguide to the detectors. The ratio fluorometer divides the red-filtered signal by the green-filtered signal, to cancel dependence on the distance (and angle) from the collection lightguide to the suspected tumor site. The ratio can be measured outside the body in a standard or phantom (a scattering and absorbing liquid approximating tissue), and the ratios compared in the body for tumors and normal tissue of the same patient. PMTs are usually used for these fluorescence power measurements. A drawback to the nonimaging method is field integration. The power measured is the integral of the fluorescence emission, including normal tissue when the tumor does not fill the field of view. Nevertheless, the ratio of red/green (R/G) has been found to complement the imaging technique if the R/G ratio is compared with the R/G ratio at a known control or nontumor site in the same patient. The latest embodiments include background subtraction and ratioing on the image, suitably coded for display of quantitative data, combining the advantages of imaging and nonimaging methods.

BIBLIOGRAPHY

Applied Optics 28(12), 15 June 1989. Special issue on tissue optics.

Boyd, R. G. 1983. *Radiometry and the detection of optical radiation*, New York: John Wiley & Sons.

Gomer, C. J., ed. 1987. *Photochemistry and Photobiology* 46(5):561–952, Nov. Special tissue on photodynamic therapy.

Hecht, E., and A. Zajac. 1976. *Optics*. Reading, Mass.: Addison-Wesley.

Hecht, J. 1986. *The laser guidebook*. New York: McGraw-Hill.

Muller, G. J., and D. H. Sliney, eds. 1989. *Dosimetry of laser radiation in medicine and biology*. Vol. IS 5, Bellingham, WA: SPIE.

O'Shea, D. C., W. R. Callen, and W. T. Rhodes. 1978. *Introduction to lasers and their applications*. Reading, Mass.: Addison-Wesley.

Profio, A. E. 1979. *Radiation shielding and dosimetry*. New York: John Wiley & Sons.

Profio, A. E. 1984. Laser excited fluorescence of hematoporphyrin derivative for diagnosis of cancer. Institute of Electrical and Electronic Engineers, *J. Quantum Electroncs* 20:1502–1507.

CHAPTER 6

RADIOLOGY

6.0 DIAGNOSTIC AND THERAPEUTIC RADIOLOGY

Diagnostic radiology is the use of radiology for diagnosis of disease or injury, based on imaging anatomical structures, including tumors, by the transmission of x-rays. The image is formed by differences in the direct transmittance, i.e., the transmittance of photons that have neither been absorbed nor scattered, and for a homogeneous medium of thickness x,

$$T = \frac{I}{I_0} = \exp(-\mu x), \tag{6.1}$$

where μ = attenuation coefficient, an energy dependent property of the medium, I is the intensity or flux measured with the body between the x-ray source and the imaging detector, and I_0 is the intensity or flux measured without the body in place. A different transmittance is measured along each ray from source to detector area (picture element or "pixel") because of differences in μ or x. If there is more than one material in the way,

$$T = \exp - (\mu_a x_1 + \mu_b x_2 + \dots), \tag{6.2}$$

where the subscripts designate the attenuation coefficient and thickness of material a or material b, etc. The geometry is shown in Fig. 6.1.

Diagnostic radiology requires a source of x-rays (collimated or small projected dimensions), an imaging detector, and an understanding of the dependence of μ on material and x-ray photon energy.

Radiotherapy, or therapeutic radiology, is concerned with depositing a

FIG. 6.1 X-ray imaging by transmittance. Ray 1 passes through the body material a with path length x_1. Ray 2 passes through an organ material b with path length x_2. The transmittance depends on the attenuation in the organ and in the body outside the organ, along ray 2 (path length approximately $x_1 - x_2$).

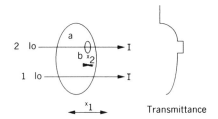

certain amount of energy per unit mass of tissue by ionization and excitation, sufficient to kill cells or at least damage them enough so that they do not reproduce. Radiotherapy is one of the main modes of cancer treatment (along with chemotherapy, conventional or laser surgery, and photodynamic therapy). The standard radiation for radiotherapy is high-energy x-rays (bremsstrahlung) from an electron accelerator such as a linac. The electrons themselves may also be used. Gamma rays from radioactive decay of radionuclides may be used instead of x-rays.

A distinction is made between teletherapy, in which the source is external to the body, and brachytherapy, in which a source of radiation is implanted interstitially or in a body cavity. The biomedical engineer or medical physicist is responsible for calibrating the source, planning the treatment procedure to deliver a prescribed dose to the tumor while sparing excessive dosing of the surrounding normal tissues, and verifying that the prescribed dose was actually delivered. It has been found that the biological effect is very sensitive to the dose, requiring precision and accuracy within a few percent. It is also necessary to limit the dose to normal tissues to avoid serious complications.

The "dose" of interest is the absorbed dose

$$D = \frac{d\varepsilon}{dm}, \tag{6.3}$$

where $d\varepsilon$ is the mean energy imparted by ionization and excitation to a mass, dm. The units of absorbed dose are thus joules per kilogram. However, the special SI unit is the gray (Gy):

$$1 \text{ Gy} = 1.0 \text{ J/kg.} \tag{6.4}$$

Formerly, the unit of absorbed dose was the rad, defined as 100 ergs per gram, hence 100 rad $=$ 1 Gy.

The attenuation of x-rays in the body is important. It must be measured or calculated to be certain the prescribed dose is delivered (e.g., to a tumor), while not exceeding a tolerable dose to the surrounding tissue. The dose should be as uniform as possible, at least within 10 percent, in the volume treated.

Radiotherapy therefore requires a source of high-energy x-rays, gamma rays, or electrons, as well as collimators and shields to define the beam in teletherapy. It is also necessary to understand the attenuation of the radiation in the body and the deposition of energy by ionization and excitation.

6.1 SOURCES

Diagnostic Radiology

The usual source of diagnostic x-rays is electron bombardment of a target, generating a continuous spectrum (bremsstrahlung) and often a line spectrum of characteristic x-rays. As shown in Fig. 6.2a, the electrons are produced by electrically heating a tungsten filament and accelerated through a potential difference up to a few hundred keV, in a vacuum, to a refractory target (usually tungsten, but may be molybdenum or another high-melting-point conductor). The target (anode) may rotate rapidly in order to spread the deposited heat over a larger area. The DC potential difference (or maximum value of a waveform with an AC component or ripple) is called kVp (kilovolt peak). Some 25 to 50 kVp is applied in mammography, and 75 to 250 kVp for thick sections or when bone intervenes, as bone has a relatively high attenuation coefficient. The electron beam current is adjustable and may range from 1 mA (for thin sections) to a few hundred mA. The exposure time is short when examining a living body, to avoid blurring from motion of the body or an organ (e.g., in respiration) and may be 0.01 to 1 second. Limiting the exposure time also alleviates the problem of dissipating heat from the anode. The x-ray apparatus is usually rated for the maximum duration of exposure, as a function of kVp and mA. Exposure time is usually specified as the product of current and exposure duration, mA-s, at a given kVp.

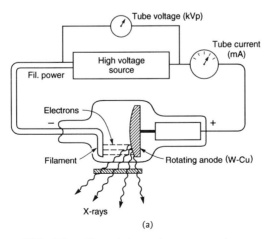

(a)

FIG. 6.2a   X-ray tube and power supply.

Radiotherapy

In radiotherapy, a high electron beam energy (on the order of 6 to 18 MeV) is used to achieve high-energy bremsstrahlung, which is attenuated only moderately in traversing the body and gives a reasonably uniform absorbed dose over several centimeters. The standard source is an electron linear accelerator, such as shown in Fig. 6.2b. The electron source is a heated cathode, and the electron beam is extracted and accelerated by a Cockcroft-Walton (CW) accelerator. Acceleration to the final voltage is achieved in the standing electromagnetic field established in a microwave waveguide by means of a klystron microwave oscillator. The waveguide is "loaded" by iris diaphragms so that the wave velocity matches the electron velocity. The klystron, and thus the electron beam, are pulsed, typically at 1 μs at 30 pulses/s. The RF buncher injects the electrons at the peak of the accelerating field. The average current may be 10 μA or so. The electron beam may emerge from the vacuum system through a thin window and may be used directly or allowed to impinge on a heavy metal target for generation of bremsstrahlung.

A typical procedure for cancer treatment consists of some 2 Gy per irradiation, repeated almost daily for a total absorbed does of some 40 to 60 Gy, depending on the type of cancer.

Radioisotopes are also used in radiotherapy. Before the introduction of the linac, a ^{60}Co gamma source of a few kilocuries was used in teletherapy. Cobalt-60 releases one 1.17-MeV gamma ray and one 1.33-MeV gamma ray per decay. These gamma rays are attenuated to about half the original intensity in about 10 cm of tissue. The source is shielded by lead, with a collimator and shutter to close of the beam between irradiations. The source to skin distance is typically 75 cm. Radioisotopes such as ^{198}Au (formerly radon) are encapsulated and inserted in the body for brachytherapy.

Superficial radiotherapy may be performed with low-energy x-rays or with high-energy electrons. With the latter, the tungsten target of the linac is

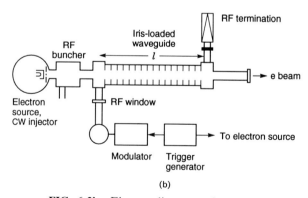

(b)

FIG. 6.2b Electron linear accelerator.

removed and replaced by a thin window for emergence of the electron beam from the vacuum system.

X-Ray Spectrum

When the energetic electrons are stopped in the target, most of the energy goes into ionization and excitation of the target atoms. This energy soon appears as heat. The rest is radiated as x-rays (bremsstrahlung or characteristic x-rays). As a rough rule of thumb, the fraction of the photon energy that appears as bremsstrahlung is

$$F_b = 10^{-6}ZV(\text{kVp}). \tag{6.5}$$

A high atomic number Z is desired as well as a high voltage. For tungsten, $Z = 74$, and about 0.007 of the energy is radiated at 100 kVp. The heating for 100 mA and 100 kVp is almost 10^4W, as so little is radiated. The process of bremsstrahlung production, illustrated in Fig. 6.3a, is deceleration of an

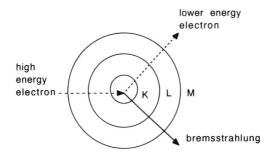

(a) generation of bremsstrahlung

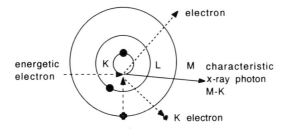

(b) generation of characteristic x-ray

FIG. 6.3 Generation of bremsstrahlung (*a*) and characteristic x-rays (*b*) by energetic electrons.

electron in the coulomb field of the nucleus. Electrons colliding with an atomic shell nucleus can eject an inner atomic electron (see Fig. 6.3b). Monoenergetic x-rays of characteristic energy are radiated as the atomic electrons cascade to lower shells. The K_α x-ray is emitted when an L-shell electron falls to the K-shell vacancy; the K_β x-ray is emitted when an M-shell electron fills the vacancy in the K-shell, and so on.

The bremsstrahlung spectrum is continuous, varying from zero intensity at the maximum energy of the incident electron (keV_{max} = kVp) to a large value at zero x-ray energy. However, the low-energy spectrum is attenuated preferentially in an x-ray tube, as well as in any "filter" or sheet of attenuating material placed at the output of the tube. Thus a typical x-ray tube spectrum appears as shown in Fig. 6.4. (for 87 kVp and a tungsten target). For tungsten, the K_α energy is 59 keV, but there is some fine structure from subshells. The spectrum also displays the K_β lines. Most of the energy goes into bremsstrahlung, rather than into characteristic x-rays. It is important to realize than the spectrum is broad and the average or "effective" energy is much less than the maximum energy (kVp), perhaps roughly half the kVp.

Low-energy x-rays are not appreciably transmitted by the body, but contribute to the radiation dose on the source side. Therefore, the x-ray tube is fitted with one or more filters (e.g., sheets of aluminum or copper) that selectively attenuate the low-energy x-rays (mostly by photoelectric effect) while transmitting most of the higher-energy x-rays. For instance, in mammography, with a compressed breast, low-energy x-rays are transmitted, but even so, some filtration is desirable.

Filtration may also be used in radiotherapy. In addition, heavy metal shields are arranged to protect organs that are not to be irradiated. A "bolus," or specially molded filter, may be arranged to make the irradiation of the tumor more uniform, e.g., by compensating for differences in thickness or geometry

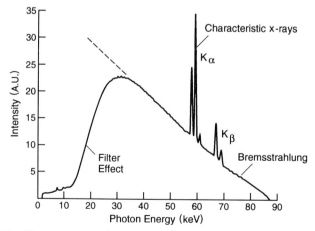

FIG. 6.4   X-ray spectrum for tungsten target, 87 kVp electrons, and filter.

near the tumor. Collimators are arranged so that the beam is shielded in all directions other than that at which the treatment volume is to be directed. In brachytherapy, the encapsulated radioactive source is not shielded, but a shielded manipulator is usually provided to protect the medical technician.

6.2 INTERACTIONS OF X-RAYS WITH MATTER

The principal interactions of x-rays with matter are (1) photoelectric effect, (2) Compton scattering, (3) pair production, and (4) Rayleigh or coherent scattering. The interactions are indicated schematically in Fig. 6.5, except for Rayleigh scattering (scattering from the whole atom), which can be disregarded in radiology.

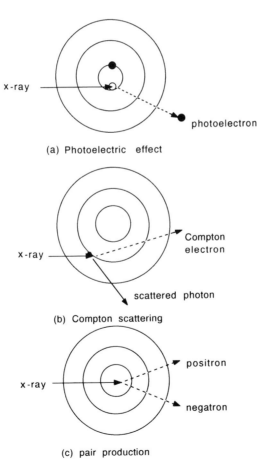

(a) Photoelectric effect

(b) Compton scattering

(c) pair production

FIG. 6.5 Interactions of x-rays with matter.

Photoelectric Effect

In the photoelectric effect, the x-ray photon is absorbed by the atom and its energy is transferred to an atomic electron. The energy of the photoelectron is

$$E_e = h\nu - E_b, \tag{6.6}$$

where $h\nu$ is the energy of the photon, and E_b is the binding energy of the electron in the atom, a function of atomic number Z. The binding energy is only a few keV or less for the elements found in the body and may be neglected for soft tissue. The attenuation coefficient is the product of the atomic density and the cross section per atom for the interaction.

$$\mu = N \frac{\text{atoms}}{\text{cm}^3} \sigma \frac{\text{cm}^2}{\text{atom}}. \tag{6.7}$$

The cross section varies as Z^4 and decreases rapidly with increasing energy, approximately as $(h\nu)^{-3}$. However, the cross section increases abruptly as the photon energy is increased above the binding energy of a group of electrons, and then decreases again as the energy is increased further. Exact values have to be obtained from a table of cross sections.

After ejection of the photoelectron, outer electrons cascade to fill the vacancy. The excess energy is dissipated by emission of monoenergetic, characteristic x-rays or low-energy electrons (Auger electrons). The ratio of characteristic x-ray photons emitted to the number of photoelectric interactions is termed the *fluorescence yield*. The fluorescence yield is very small for low Z atoms. In any case, the low-energy x-rays and Auger electrons are insignificant in radiology.

Compton Scattering

Compton scattering involves scattering from a "free" electron, i.e., an electron in an atom whose binding energy is small as compared with the photon energy. The interaction may be analyzed as a two-body elastic collision between photon and electron at rest, taking into account relativistic effects. The energy of the Compton electron is

$$E_e = \frac{h\nu\alpha(1 - \cos\theta)}{[1 + \alpha(1 - \cos\theta)]}, \tag{6.8}$$

where $\alpha = h\nu/m_0c^2 = h\nu/511$ keV, and θ is the angle between the directions of the scattered and incident photons. The maximum energy occurs for scattering through π radians or 180° and gives the energy of the "Compton edge" or

$$E_{max} = \frac{h\nu}{[1 + (1/2\alpha)]} \qquad (6.9)$$

The energy of the Compton-scattered photon is

$$h\nu' = \frac{h\nu}{[1 + \alpha(1 - \cos \theta)]} . \qquad (6.10)$$

The angular distribution of the scattered photon is given by the Klein-Nishina formula, plotted in Fig. 6.6 for several values of the photon energy. The mass absorption coefficient (μ/p) is a function of energy as shown in Fig. 6.7 and varies as $Z\sigma_e$, where σ_e is the Compton cross section per electron, 0.665×10^{-24} cm². This figure also plots the mass attenuation coefficients for the photoelectric effect and for pair production, in water, which is similar to tissue in attenuation.

Pair Production

In pair production, the x-ray disappears and two electrons are created, one with a positive charge (positron) and one with a negative charge (negatron). The positron soon slows to low energies and reacts with the negatron (e.g., atomic electron), releasing two annihilation quanta (gamma rays), each of 511 keV energy. The total energy shared by the positron and the negatron is equal to the energy of the x-ray, but as $2m_0c^2 = 1022$ keV, and the rest energies of two electrons is required to create the electrons, and the kinetic energy shared between them is only

$$E_{e+,e-} = h\nu - 1022 \text{ keV} \qquad (6.11)$$

The cross section is proportional to Z^2, but zero below 1022 keV and increases only slowly with photon energy. Pair production is zero in diagnostic radiology and is often ignored in radiotherapy of tissue, even with a source energy above 1022 keV.

Total Attenuation Coefficient

The total attenuation coefficient, or just attenuation coefficient, is equal to the sum of the attenuation coefficients for the various interactions and summed over the elements in the tissue:

$$\mu = \Sigma_i(\mu_{pei} + \mu_{cei} + \mu_{ppi}) \qquad (6.12)$$

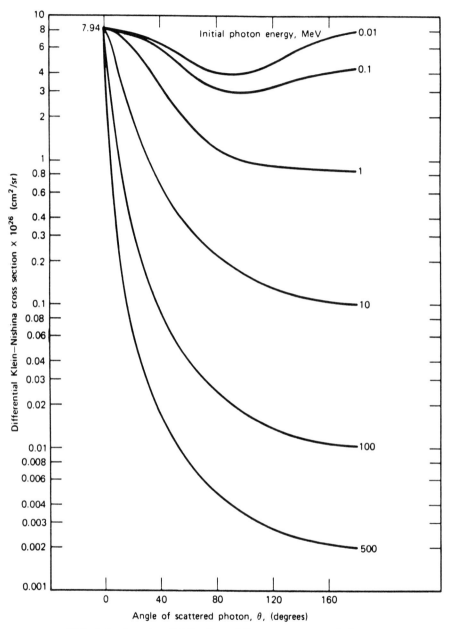

FIG. 6.6 Angular distribution of Compton-scattered photons.

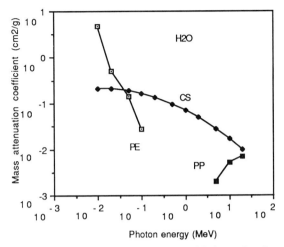

FIG. 6.7 Photoelectric (PE), Compton scattering (CS), and pair production (PP) mass attenuation coefficients (cm^2/g) for water as a function of photon energy (MeV).

The attenuation coefficient may be expressed in terms of the linear attenuation coefficient $\mu(cm^{-1})$, in which case the thickness of tissue is expressed as $x(cm)$, or by the mass attenuation coefficient (μ/ρ) (cm^2/g) with the thickness expressed as ρx (g/cm^2). The latter is plotted for muscle and bone, in Fig. 6.8. The mass coefficient of body tissues is essentially independent of energy above about 100 keV, reflecting the dominance of Compton scattering (because the

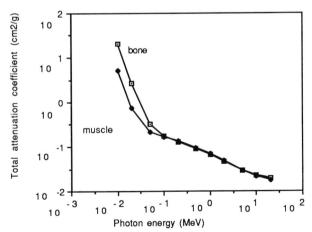

FIG. 6.8 Total mass attenuation coefficient (cm^2/g) vs. photon energy (MeV) for compact bone and striated muscle. (Data from J. H. Hubbell, "Photon Cross Sections, Attenuation Coefficients, and Energy Absorption Coefficients from 10 keV to 100 GeV," Report NSRDS-NBS 29 (1969), Sup. Documents, U.S. Govt. Printing Office, Washington, DC.

Compton scattering coefficient is proportional to electron density, which is approximately proportional to mass density for most elements other than hydrogen). If the contrast is too low, it can be increased by administering a contrast agent that has a high Z or density. Common contrast agents include solutions of an iodine compound, often misnamed a "dye," (for imaging blood vessels, for example) and barium sulfate (an insoluble compound that fills or coats the wall of the digestive tract when swallowed.

Mass interaction coefficients and the mass energy absorption coefficient are given in Table 6.1 for water (similar to tissue), from 0.01 to 10 or 20 MeV. The photoelectric (pe), Compton scattering (cs), pair production (pp) and total (t) coefficients are listed. The mass energy absorption coefficient, μ_{en}/ρ, refers to the energy transferred to electrons, and the energy deposited in the material by excitation and ionization. It includes essentially all of the x-ray energy transferred to electrons by the photoelectric effect (assuming

TABLE 6.1   Mass Attenuation and Energy Deposition Coefficients (cm^2/g) for Water

E (MeV)	μ_{pe}/ρ	μ_{cs}/ρ	μ_{pp}/ρ	μ_t/ρ	μ_{en}/ρ
0.01	4.78	0.214		4.99	4.79
0.015	1.27	0.210		1.48	1.28
0.02	0.505	0.207		0.711	0.512
0.03	0.138	0.200		0.338	0.149
0.04	0.055	0.193		0.248	0.0678
0.05	0.027	0.188		0.214	0.0419
0.06	0.015	0.182		0.197	0.0320
0.08	0.006	0.173		0.179	0.0262
0.10	0.003	0.165		0.168	0.0256
0.15	0.001	0.148		0.149	0.0277
0.20	0.000	0.136		0.136	0.0297
0.03		0.118		0.118	0.0319
0.40		0.106		0.106	0.0328
0.50		0.097		0.097	0.0330
0.60		0.090		0.090	0.0329
0.80		0.079		0.079	0.0321
1.00		0.071		0.071	0.0309
1.50		0.057	0.000	0.057	0.0282
2.00		0.049	0.000	0.049	0.0260
3.00		0.038	0.001	0.039	0.0227
4.00		0.032	0.002	0.034	0.0206
5.00		0.028	0.002	0.030	0.0191
6.00		0.024	0.003	0.027	0.0180
8.00		0.020	0.004	0.024	0.0166
10.00		0.017	0.005	0.022	0.0157
15.00		0.013	0.006	0.019	—
20.00		0.010	0.007	0.017	—

the characteristic x-rays are reabsorbed), the energy of the Compton electron, and the kinetic energy imparted to the negatron and positron in pair production. However, this energy is the x-ray photon energy less the mass-energy 1.022 MeV, which may or may not be reabsorbed because the annihilation quanta may escape. Losses from bremsstrahlung from the secondary electrons have to be taken into account as well.

6.3   X-RAY TRANSPORT

Diagnostic Radiology

The x-ray image is generated by the uncollided photons (those that have been neither scattered nor absorbed). For a point isotropic source, the photon flux density (photons/cm²s) varies as $1/r^2$ at distance r from the source, and exponentially because of the interactions in a thickness x of material between source and detector:

$$\Phi = \frac{S}{4\pi r^2} \exp(-\mu x), \tag{6.13}$$

where S is the source strength (photons/s) and μ is the total attenuation coefficient (cm-1).

The main problems in x-ray transport in diagnostic radiology are to approximate a point source and to avoid detection of scattered photons. The electron spot on the target of the x-ray tube is made small, e.g., with projected dimensions of about 1 to 3 mm. Even so, the image will have a penumbra, or partial shadow, as shown in Fig. 6.9. To reduce the penumbra, the source

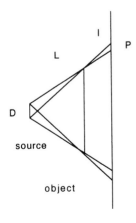

FIG. 6.9   Penumbra from finite area x-ray source. D is the diameter of the source, L the source-object distance, l the object-film distance, and P the width of the penumbra. Then $P = D(l/L)$.

size should be minimized, the distance between source and object maximized, and the distance from object to detector (such as film) minimized.

If the detector output is a function of energy, e.g., a scintillation detector, it may be possible to discriminate against scattered photons because their energy will be lower than the uncollided source photons. With a broad-spectrum x-ray source, however, this is not practical. In any case, film does not provide energy information. Instead, a Bucky-Potter grid or multihole collimator is used between the object and the film, such as shown in Fig. 6.10. The grid is oscillated to avoid leaving an image of the grid on the film. X-rays that pass between the lead strips are imaged, whereas scattered x-rays strike the sides of the lead strips and are absorbed. The Bucky-Potter grid is often used in imaging the abdomen because of the large scattering in this thick and dense body section. The price is a reduction in sensitivity, as some of the x-rays are absorbed in the grid.

A disadvantage of conventional x-ray imaging is that the roentgengram is a two-dimensional projection of a three-dimensional object. Structures above and below the desired plane overlap. This problem is solved by computed tomography (CT), discussed later.

Radiotherapy

The transport of x-rays is governed by the Boltzmann transport equation and may be calculated by the same computer methods used for the transport of light, e.g., discrete ordinates or Monte Carlo. A complication is the change in energy as well as direction in Compton scattering. In the discrete ordinates method, it is usual to divide the energy into contiguous intervals or groups, with the cross sections or attenuation coefficients being averages over the interval. The angular distribution of scattering, $S(\theta)$, is usually represented as the sum of terms involving coefficients times Legendre polynomials in the

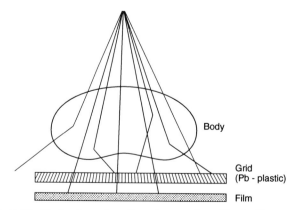

FIG. 6.10 Reduction of scattered x-rays by a Bucky-Potter grid.

cosine of the scattering angle, i.e., $\chi = \cos \theta$. The first few Legendre polynomials are the following:

$$P_0(\chi) = 1$$
$$P_1(\chi) = \chi$$
$$P_2(\chi) = 0.5(3\chi^2 - 1)$$
$$P_3(\chi) = 0.5(5\chi^3 - 3\chi)$$

In Monte Carlo, it is not necessary to use groups, except perhaps when the scores are calculated. Likewise, the angular distribution of scattering may use the Legendre polynomial expansion or the direct $S(\theta)$. The energy $E = h\nu$ of the scattered photon is related to θ and the energy of the incident photon by equation 6.10.

The attentuation of uncollided photons is exponential, so a plot of the natural logarithm of the photon flux density versus distance in an attenuator is a straight line, as shown in Fig. 6.11. Some of the scattered photons make multiple scatters and again contribute to the main beam. Under certain conditions, there is a buildup near the source, as seen in Fig. 6.11, and then a more or less exponential drop-off with distance, which is, however, slower than for the uncollided flux density.

Measurement

The photon flux density and its spectrum are seldom measured, because the main interest is in the dose. However, the flux density spectrum can be measured with either a thallium-activated scintillation detector, NaI(Tl), or a silicon or germanium diode. The scintillation detector consists of a NaI(Tl) crystal in a light-tight case (except for a window at one end) with white diffuse reflector coating on the inside of the case, optically coupled through an index-matching silicone gel to the faceplate of an end window photomultiplier tube. The scintillation crystal emits a weak flash of light when excited by a secondary electron from x-ray or γ-ray interactions. The light releases photoelectrons, and the photoelectron current pulse is amplified by the electron multiplier and then generates a voltage pulse across the anode load resistor. The voltage

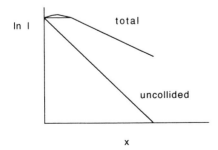

FIG. 6.11   Attenuation of uncollided photons and uncollided plus scattered photons.

pulse is amplified and shaped by an electronic, usually transistor, amplifier. The amplitude of the voltage pulse (maximum voltage) is nearly proportional to the energy deposited in the crystal by x-ray or γ-ray interactions, whereas the number of pulses (counts) per second is a measure of the number of photons incident.

In the silicon or germanium detector, a crystal of very pure Si or Ge is doped to form a p-n junction diode. If the requisite purity cannot be obtained, the effect of impurities can be canceled by drifting lithium into the proper region, hence the Si(Li) and Ge(Li) diodes. The p-n junction is reverse-biased at a couple thousand volts, forming a "depletion region," which is the sensitive volume. Electrons and holes released by secondary electrons from x-ray or γ-ray interactions are collected and amplified to give a voltage pulse whose amplitude is proportional to the energy deposited in the sensitive volume. Both Si(Li) and Ge(Li) detectors are refrigerated to 77K, the liquid nitrogen boiling point, to reduce noise and prevent rediffusion of the Li, hence they must also be stored at 77K. The high-purity Ge detector, HPGe, does not require Li and may be stored at room temperature. It must, however, also be operated at 77K.

The spectral flux density can be unfolded from the response functions (counts/s vs. amplitude calibrated in terms of energy). Figure 6.12 plots the response functions for several gamma rays from radioactive sources. The

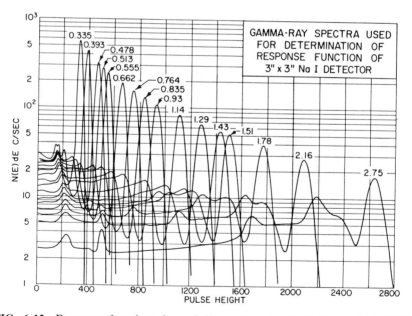

FIG. 6.12 Response functions for a 7.62 cm diameter by 7.62 cm thick NaI(Tl) scintillator at several gamma ray energies (MeV). (From R. L. Heath, Report "Scintillation Spectrometry Gamma Ray Spectrum Catalog," 2nd Ed., Report IDO-16880-1 (1964). Dept. of Energy Technical Document.

response functions at intermediate energies can be found by interpolation. There are computer programs to unfold the flux density spectrum from a measured count rate versus energy spectrum, given the response functions.

6.4 IMAGING DETECTORS

Film-Screen

The standard imaging detector for x-rays is film (a relatively thick layer, on the order of 10 μm, of silver halide and gelatin emulsion coated on both sides of a transparent plastic sheet). The film may be used alone or sandwiched between intensifying screens. These are sheets coated with a phosphor that absorbs some of the x-rays and emits light. When exposed to x-rays or light, the film forms a latent image that is made visible by the usual chemical processing. A developer reduces the activated silver halide to fine particles of metallic silver (appearing black). A fixing solution removes the remaining silver halide, and then the film is washed and dried. Because processing of medical roentgengrams is now done in automatic machines, a darkroom and manual handling are not needed.

In most diagnostic radiology, the negative is used. Therefore, a region of low x-ray attenuation results in more x-rays reaching the film, and the developed film appears dark in that region. The projected image of bone appears more or less transparent, because few x-rays penetrate the bone and expose the film. To prevent exposure to light, the film is enclosed in a cassette or holder that is transparent to x-rays but opaque to visible light.

To reduce the exposure (J/cm^2) required to activate the silver halide (and hence the dose to the patient), the double-coated film may be sandwiched between thin (on the order of 100 μm) sheets coated with a fluorescent compound such as calcium tungstate. The film and screens are held in intimate contact by evacuating the cassette, or by the pressure of a compressible sheet. The x-rays interact with the fluorescent substance (preferably one containing high Z elements for increased photoelectric effect and absorption coefficient). The light emitted as fluorescence then exposes the film as in photography. The most efficient screens, and thus the lowest dose, are achieved with fluorescent compounds (phosphors) of rare earth elements. A disadvantage of screens is the diffusion of light in them, resulting in a roentgengram not quite as sharp as with film alone.

The contrast characteristics of a given film-screen combination are presented in the Hurter-Driffield or characteristic curve, such as shown in Fig. 6.13. The abscissa is the logarithm of the x-ray exposure (J/cm^2, for example). The ordinate is the diffuse optical density of the developed film:

$$OD = \log \frac{I_0}{I},$$

$$(6.14)$$

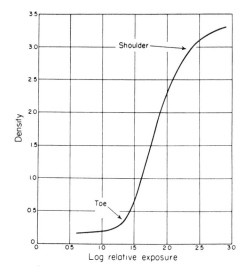

FIG. 6.13 Characteristic curve of an x-ray film with $CaWO_4$ intensifying screen.

where I_0 is the densitometer signal without the film, and I is the signal with the film between the lamp and the diffusor-equipped photodetector. There is a region where OD versus log exposure is more or less linear. The slope is large for "fast" films and small for "slow" films. A fast film reaches a usable OD at lower exposure than a slow film, and the contrast is greater (larger difference in OD for a given difference in exposure, such as experienced when comparing adjacent regions of slightly different attenuation). On the other hand, the fast film has a smaller "latitude," or difference in log exposure over the usable range of OD. The characteristic curve has a "toe" corresponding to a region where the base fog is significant (the background OD from the film sheet and natural exposure). There is a "shoulder" and a nonlinear region at large exposures. The latitude is usually defined for an exposure giving an OD of 1.0 above base fog, to the exposure at the start of the shoulder. The usable OD range is limited at the high-exposure end by the shoulder or by a density so great that small differences cannot be perceived by the eye when the film is mounted on a light box (a diffusing glass uniformly backlit by a number of fluorescent tubes). The characteristic curve is measured by irradiating a step-wedge placed on the film. The step-wedge is made like a staircase, in that the thickness of the wedge is made to vary in a steplike fashion. The OD for each thickness is measured after processing, whereas the log exposure follows from the exposure with no material and the attenuation factor corresponding to each step thickness.

Besides contrast, the film or film-screen combination has to provide a reasonable spatial resolution. Resolution may be specified in terms of line-pairs per millimeter: the number of pairs of opaque and transmitting lines, per millimeter that can just be discerned in the image. It can be measured by placing a target with x-ray attenuating and transmitting strips on the film. Another measure is the "unsharpness," or width of the blurred region at an edge where theoretically the OD should change abruptly between two values (corresponding to an edge in attenuation, and hence exposure). For film without screens, the unsharpness is very small (on the order of 1 μm). Because of the spreading and scattering of the fluorescent light in an intensifying screen, the unsharpness is greater (on the order of 100 μm).

Xerographic Plate

Xerography may be applied to imaging x-rays, especially the low-voltage x-rays (on the order of 50 kVp) used in examination of the breast (xeromammography). The imaging detector is a positively charged selenium-coated plate. Selenium is a semiconductor. When exposed to x-rays, the selenium is made conductive and some of the charge leaks off. The greater the exposure in a region, the lower the charge remaining. The image is made visible by dusting the plate with negatively charged powder (usually plastic microspheres dyed blue), as shown in Fig. 6.14. More powder is attracted to the more positively charged areas in the selenium plate. The image is transferred to white paper, and the powder (toner) is fused to the paper by heat. The final result is a positive "print" viewed in reflected light. The selenium plate is cleaned and reused. With this method, the dose to the patient is larger than with film-screen radiography.

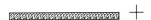 +

(a) Positively-charged Se plate

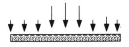

(b) Exposed to x-rays. Charge leaks according to x-ray intensity.

(c) Dusted with negatively-charged powder. More powder retained where charge is greater.

FIG. 6.14 Principle of xeroradiography.

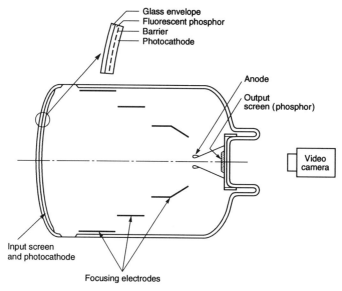

FIG. 6.15 Image intensifier and video camera for x-ray fluoroscopy. X-rays produce light in fluorescent phosphor, which releases electrons from the photocathode. Electrons are accelerated and focused on the output screen. The image is viewed by the video camera.

Fluoroscope

X-rays can be imaged by the light emitted from a scintillation crystal that is thick enough to have a reasonable detection efficiency and thin enough that spreading of light is not too great (although the spatial resolution is not as good as can be obtained by film). The weak scintillation light is detected and amplified by an image intensifier. The output of the intensifier is a phosphor viewed by a sensitive video camera. The scintillator and intensifier photocathode have to be large enough to cover the entire area of interest. A typical image intensifier with an integral scintillator (fluorescent layer) is shown in Fig. 6.15. This tube demagnifies the image, increasing brightness and easing optical coupling to the video camera. Fluoroscopy is used when it is important to examine organs in motion or in real time, without the delay associated with exposure and processing of film or a selenium plate. The dose to the patient, however, is often high as compared with the dose in film or film-screen radiography or in xeroradiography.

6.5 COMPUTED TOMOGRAPHY

CT is a revolutionary development in diagnostic radiology. It images a layer in the body, which is usually perpendicular to the long axis of the body (hence its former name, computerized axial tomography [CAT]). There is no blurring resulting from the superposition of overlying or underlying structures. Accurate quantitative measurements of the total attenuation coefficient versus position are obtained, which helps to distinguish one tissue from another. On the other hand, resolution (approximately 5 mm by 5 mm by 10 mm thickness of the layer) is not as good as with regular x-ray images. The derivation of the attenuation coefficients from measured transmittances requires a computer, hence the name *computed tomography*. Because the imaging detector is an array of collimated scintillation counters and the x-ray beam is collimated, there is less scattering than with conventional radiology.

CT Scanners

The principle of a CT scanner is diagrammed in Fig. 6.16. The layer is in the plane of the paper. An x-ray source and small scintillation detector define a line through the body in the transverse plane. The transmittance of x-ray is measured. Then the source and detector are scanned (translated) another step, definining another path through the body, parallel to the first. The process is repeated until the entire body section has been scanned. The "absorption profile" in Fig. 6.16 is a plot of the absorptance $(1 - \text{transmittance})$ as a function of position in the translation direction. At any one position, the transmittance follows the exponential function (see equation 6.2), where the sum is for all materials along the ray between source and detector. Yet this information alone is not sufficient to define the attenuation coefficients μ_i. Instead, the entire mechanism for linear translation of source and detector is rotated through a certain angle, and another linear traverse is taken. In Fig. 6.16, only two angles are shown at 0° and 90°. In practice, the increment

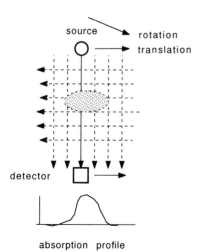

absorption profile

FIG. 6.16 Principle of computed tomography with translating and rotating source-detector.

in angle is small, perhaps 1°, giving some 180 angles altogether. If the step in translation is, for instance, 5 mm, and the length of the traverse is 300 mm, then $60 \times 180 = 1.08 \times 10^4$ measured transmittances are obtained. A computer algorithm is required to unfold a matrix of attenuation coefficient versus position from the transmittances. The thicknesses (at a given angle) are all the same, defined by the computational matrix which in turn is related to resolution afforded by the x-ray beam width and detector dimensions. For example, with 5 mm $\times$ 5 mm cells, and a 300 mm $\times$ 300 mm overall field, the attenuation coefficient is desired in each of $60 \times 60 = 3.6 \times 10^3$ squares.

The source in CT is the usual x-ray tube. The operating voltage may be about 150 kVp. The detector is a scintillation counter sensitive to the x-ray energies of interest. To save space and still maintain good detection efficiency, the original sodium iodide scintillator is being replaced by bismuth germanate (BGO), even though its light output is much less. The detector is usually operated in the current rather than the pulse mode, because of the large dynamic range and the high number of events detected in the short time available before the detector is scanned to a new position. Actually, in the latest version of CT machines, the scanned detector is replaced by a stationary array of detectors, and the x-ray source is applied in fan beam geometry, as shown in Fig. 6.17. In the third-generation machines, both x-ray source and detector array are rotated together to generate data at many angles. In the fourth-generation machines, the detector array is a circle, only the x-ray source is rotated (inside the circle), and the proper angles and positions are obtained electronically.

The dimensions of all pixels are the same, thus only the attenuation coefficient is needed. The transmittances are measured to 0.1 percent, and the unfolded attenuation coefficient is obtained to within 5 percent. A complication with the broad spectrum produced by an x-ray tube is "beam hardening." The lower-energy x-rays are attenuated more than the higher-energy x-rays, so that the spectrum shifts to a higher average energy, dependent on the thickness traveled in the body; therefore, the attenuation coefficient varies with position. In the first machines, for imaging the head, a water-filled bag

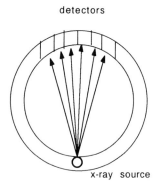

FIG. 6.17 Fan beam geometry with multiple detectors. Assembly is rotated.

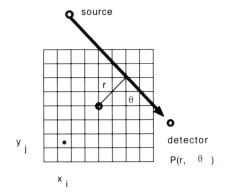

FIG. 6.18 Geometry for image reconstruction. Obtain attenuation coefficient μ_{ij} in pixel x_iy_j by unfolding absorption profile at many angles, or from $P(r, \theta)$ for ray at radius r and angle θ to x-axis.

was placed around the head to compensate for this artifact. In later machines, the beam-hardening correction is calculated from the geometry or from a calibration experiment.

Unfolding Methods

The unfolding or reconstruction of the pattern of attenuation coefficients from the measured transmittances or "line integral values" or "ray sums" is the heart of CT. The Austrian mathematician Radon proved the existence of such an unfolded solution. Reduction to a useful clinical instrument (initially for the head) was the accomplishment of the British computer scientist Hounsfield and the engineers of EMI, Ltd.

The reconstruction geometry is shown in Fig. 6.18. The attenuation coefficients are to be calculated for $i \times j$ pixels of the same size in a square map, from the measured ray sums at various angles θ and positions that can be denoted by the radius r. In discrete form,

$$P_j = \Sigma_i W_{i,j} U(i), \qquad (6.15)$$

where P_j is the ith ray sum or "projection" ($j = 1$ to M). The sum is over $i = 1$ to N. W is a weighting function. $U(i)$ is the attenuation coefficient, and i indexes all points (x, y). W is zero if no rays intersect for i and j. Otherwise, it is related to the path length through the cell or pixel square. The inverse problem (unfolding) is to solve for $U(i)$. Several methods have been devised to do this by computer:

1. Summation methods (e.g., simple back projection)
2. Transform methods (e.g., Fourier transform)
3. Direct analytic methods (e.g., convolution, filtered back projection)
4. Iterative methods.

The simple back projection is shown in Fig. 6.19. For M values of projection P_j, the simple back projection for each pixel gives

$$U(i) = \Sigma_j P_j \cdot K_{i,j} \qquad (i = 1, N)(j = 1, M), \qquad (6.16)$$

where $K_{i,j}$ is a special weighting function equal to zero if ray j does not intersect pixel i, and equal to 1 if it does. As can be seen from the Fig. 6.19, the reconstructed image of a circular object shows a star pattern, or in the limit of many angles, a blurred edge. Simple back projection is not satisfactory.

The Fourier-transform technique requires transformation of the projection profiles into Fourier space (spatial frequencies instead of positions), application of a mathematical filtering function, and transforming back into the spatial domain to provide an estimate of the object.

The most common method is the convolution or filtered back projection (FBP), which is based on the Fourier method. Figure 6.20 shows a filter function (termed Ram-Lak) used with FBP. The method is illustrated in Fig. 6.21. It is similar to simple back projection except for the (spatial domain) filter function, which has the effect of removing the "star" pattern or halo of decreasing density around an object.

An example of the iterative technique is shown in Fig. 6.22. The technique is based on an initial estimate of the attenuation coefficient in each pixel. Then new ray sums are calculated and compared with actual ray sums. The difference is reduced by either a multiplicative or an additive factor, and the process is continued until the difference between calculated and measured ray sums is small enough to be negligible. The example is for a two-by-two

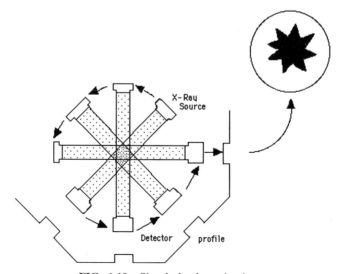

FIG. 6.19 Simple back projection.

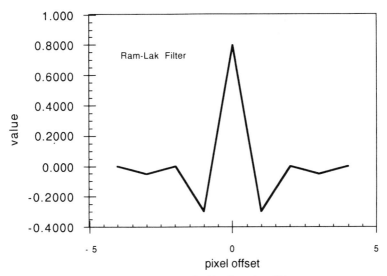

FIG. 6.20 "Ram-Lak" filter for CT.

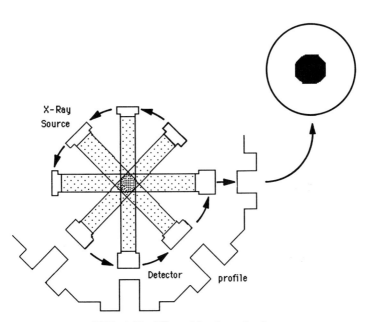

FIG. 6.21 Filtered back projection.

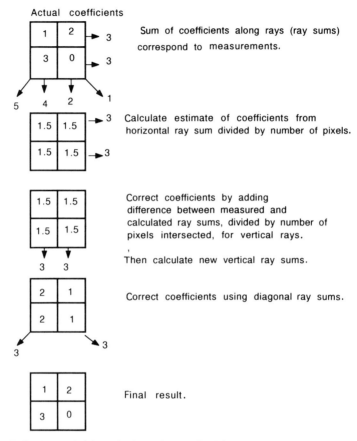

Actual coefficients

Sum of coefficients along rays (ray sums) correspond to measurements.

Calculate estimate of coefficients from horizontal ray sum divided by number of pixels.

Correct coefficients by adding difference between measured and calculated ray sums, divided by number of pixels intersected, for vertical rays.

Then calculate new vertical ray sums.

Correct coefficients using diagonal ray sums.

Final result.

FIG. 6.22 Arithmetic, iterative method for image reconstruction.

array of pixels, with 6 rays. In CT, there will be hundreds or thousands of pixels and projections, and a computer is needed to carry out the calculations.

Quantitative Image

One of the great advantages of CT is its ability to measure and distinguish quite small differences in attenuation coefficient, and hence tissue density and composition. It is convenient to normalize to the attenuation coefficient of water, μ_w, giving a "CT number" or "Hounsfield number":

$$H = \frac{1000(\mu - \mu_w)}{\mu_w} \qquad (6.17)$$

Tissues with attenuation coefficients less than the attenuation coefficient of water have H between 0 and -1000. Tissues with higher attenuation coef-

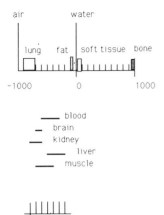

air   water

lung   fat soft tissue bone

-1000   0   1000

___ blood
_   brain
___ kidney
    ___ liver
  ___ muscle

|||||||
20   80

FIG. 6.23 Attenuation coefficient in terms of Hounsfield number, for various tissues.

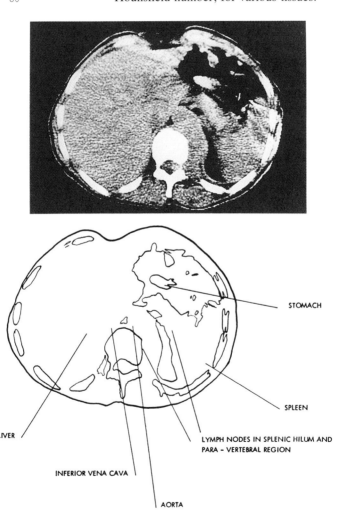

STOMACH

SPLEEN

LIVER

LYMPH NODES IN SPLENIC HILUM AND
PARA - VERTEBRAL REGION

INFERIOR VENA CAVA

AORTA

FIG. 6.24 Computed tomography scan through abdomen. (Courtesy of J. R. Cameron, University of Wisconsin, Madison.)

ficients have H between 0 and $+1000$. Actual resolution is a few Hounsfield units. As indicated in Fig. 6.23, soft tissues vary from about $H = 20$ to 80, for the 72 keV effective energy. Fat is less attenuating and varies from about $H = -70$ to $H = -100$. Lungs are of low density because of the air, and H varies from about -750 to -900. CT images, such as shown in Fig. 6.24, use a gray scale and may shift the gray tone assigned to to H = 0 and expand the span of gray tones displayed for a given span of input H values to make subtle differences more easily seen. Contrast media may be used to increase contrast when necessary.

6.6 DOSIMETRY

The desired quantity in radiotherapy, absorbed dose, may be calculated or measured. Actually, one calculates the Kerma (kinetic energy released in material) by

$$K = \frac{dE_K}{dm} = \left(\frac{\mu_{en}}{\rho}\right)\Phi , \tag{6.18}$$

where dE_K is the kinetic energy of charged particles (e.g., electrons) released by indirectly ionizing radiation (e.g., x-rays, gamma rays) in a tissue mass dm, and (μ_{en}/ρ) is the mass energy transfer coefficient averaged over the spectrum of the particle fluence Φ. For x-rays or gamma rays, the energy transfer includes the energy of the photoelectron, the average energy of the Compton electron, and the kinetic energies of the positron and negatron in pair production. The ratio of x-ray fluence to Kerma is plotted as a function of energy in Fig. 6.25, for bone and for muscle. Values of μ_{en}/ρ from 10 keV to 10 MeV are listed in Table 6.1 for water, which is close to soft tissue.

The significance of Kerma is that it can be equated to absorbed dose under certain circumstances. The conditions of radiation and charged-particle (electron) equilibrium must be achieved. In radiation equilibrium, energy leaving a differential volume of mass (dm) (far from the boundaries) is compensated for by energy entering the volume, and the condition implies a more or less uniform radiation field. Under conditions of charged-particle equilibrium (c.p.e.), a charged particle carrying a given energy away from the differential volume is compensated for by another charged particle of equal energy. C.p.e. is expected to break down at high energies, near a point source or near boundaries. Nevertheless, c.p.e. is often assumed or arranged in both calculations and measurements because a direct determination of absorbed dose is difficult.

Another complication is bremsstrahlung produced by the charged particles. This energy is included in Kerma but is missing from the absorbed dose because the bremsstrahlung will escape from the vicinity of the dose point.

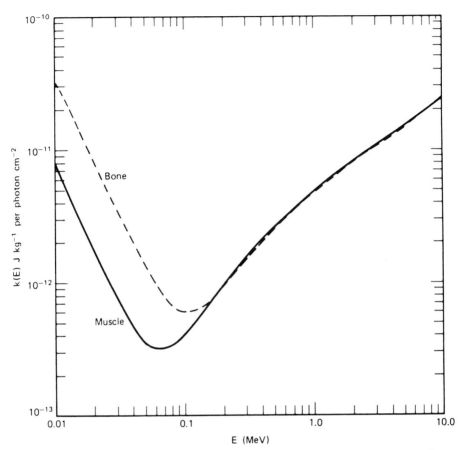

FIG. 6.25 Ratio of Kerma to gamma or x-ray fluence vs. energy. (From Profio, A. E. 1979. *Radiation shielding and dosimetry*. New York: John Wiley & Sons.)

Often bremsstrahlung is small for the low atomic number elements in soft tissue and may be ignored. If not, the generation and transport of bremsstrahlung must be included in the calculations and a correction made to convert Kerma to absorbed dose. An example of the variation of Kerma and absorbed dose with depth in muscle and bone is shown schematically in Fig. 6.26. Note that the absorbed dose is lower at the surface than inside the muscle (or other tissue) because of backscattering. This reduction of dose at the surface is important in skin sparing: the skin is radiosensitive and the reduction in dose in and near the skin reduces the side effects of radiotherapy.

Calculation of Dose

The transport of ionizing radiation is described by the Boltzmann equation, which can be solved, subject to the boundary conditions, by the discrete

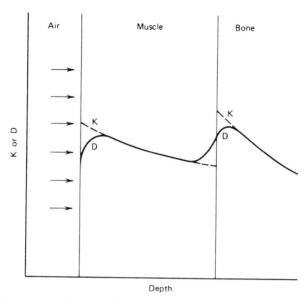

FIG. 6.26 Variation of Kerma (K) and absorbed dose (D) with depth for x-rays perpendicularly incident on muscle from air. Note the buildup of D as electrons attain equilibrium in muscle, and the larger D in bone and muscle near bone.

ordinates method discussed in Chapter 5. The spatial and spectral distribution of the radiant energy fluence rate, F(r, E), can also be calculated by the Monte Carlo method (see Chapter 5). Diffusion theory is not a good approximation for high-energy x-rays or gamma rays or fast neutrons because of the anisotropic scattering. The absorbed dose or Kerma has to be calculated for complex geometries in the individual patient. Because a complete calculation can take a long time with use of a large high-speed computer, a medium-speed minicomputer is often used to combine previously calculated solutions, for instance, by superposition of sources, with spectra as a function of depth in a homogeneous medium away from boundaries. The treatment planner has to describe the organ type, position, and boundaries, perhaps from a CT scan. He or she also proposes one or several beam geometries and intensities for a trial plan, modifying it as necessary to achieve the desired uniformity of dose while sparing radiosensitive normal tissues.

Measurement of Dose

The absorbed dose is usually measured by an ionization chamber such as shown in Fig. 6.27 or a smaller one. The walls and electrode are made of a tissue-equivalent plastic (one that contains the same principal elements and proportions as soft tissue, $C_5H_{40}O_{18}N$). The cavity is filled with a tissue-

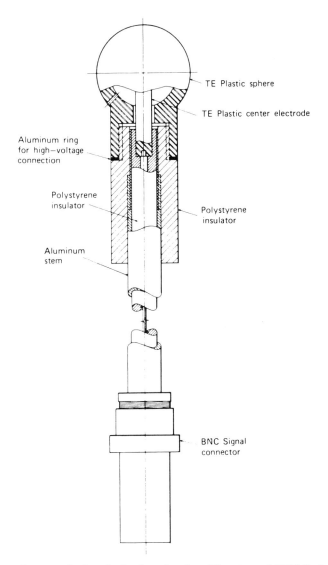

FIG. 6.27 Tissue equivalent ionization chamber (Courtesy of EG&G, Inc., Goleta, CA.)

equivalent gas (e.g., 64.4 vol. percent CH_4, 32.4 vol. percent CO_2, and 3.2 vol. percent N_2). The walls are made thick enough for c.p.e. (thicker than the range of the most energetic electrons), but no thicker, to avoid attenuation of the x-rays or gamma rays. Figure 6.27 shows an ionization chamber with walls 5 mm thick, and a gas volume of 1 cm^3 at 1 atm pressure. The DC potential across the gas space is 250 V.

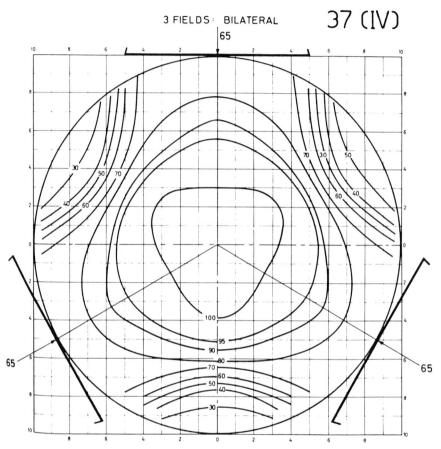

FIG. 6.28 Isodose curves for irradiation at three angles with a ^{60}Co gamma ray teletherapy source. (From M. Cohen and S. J. Martin. 1966. *Atlas of radiation dose distributions*. Vol. 2. Vienna: IAEA.)

The energy absorbed per gram of gas is

$$D_c = WJ_m, \tag{6.19}$$

where W is the energy per ion pair in the filling gas (typically around 30 eV), and J_m is the measured number of ion pairs (from the charge collected) per gram of gas. According to Bragg-Gray cavity ionization chamber theory, the energy absorbed per gram in the wall,

$$D_w = s_m D_c, \tag{6.20}$$

where s_m is the ratio of the stopping power in the wall to the stopping power in the gas. If both are the same composition (tissue equivalent), the ratio is unity. The chamber design assumes c.p.e., a nonperturbing cavity, and that essentially all electrons originate in the wall. The dimensions of the cavity are small as compared with the range of the electrons at the gas pressure used. The absorbed dose in the wall is then a good approximation of the absorbed dose in soft tissue.

Dose Distribution

The spatial distribution of an absorbed dose may be measured by moving the ionization chamber in a phantom (water, or better tissue-equivalent liquid or plastic), with the same beam or source geometry as will be used in the actual irradiation. It is standard practice to plot the isodose curves so derived, connecting points of the same dose. The isodose chart usually plots a cross section through the beam axis or source. To avoid radiosensitive structures and improve uniformity of irradiation of the tumor, the tumor may be placed at the intersection of perhaps, three beams, as shown in Fig. 6.28. The patient remains in a fixed position while the cobalt-60, linac, or other source is rotated so that an irradiation is performed at each of three angles. The tumor receives three doses, whereas most of the tissue receives only one dose.

In brachytherapy, the radioactive source is implanted in a body cavity or even interstitially. Again, isodose curves may be measured or calculated. The decrease with distance from the source is more rapid in brachytherapy than in teletherapy.

6.7 OER AND RBE

The absorbed dose is not the only determinant of the biological effect. The effect depends on the density of ionizations along the path (linear energy transfer [LET]), hence the type of ionizing charged particle, and for low LET, the pressure or concentration of molecular oxygen in the tissue.

Low-LET radiation (x-rays and electrons) in tissue, which is some 80 percent water, acts mostly indirectly through production of free radicals.

$$H_2O \rightarrow H_2O^+ + e^- \quad \text{(ionization)}$$

$$H_2O^+ \rightarrow H^+ + OH^0 \quad \text{(hydroxyl radical)}$$

$$H_2O + e^- \rightarrow OH^- + H^0 \quad \text{(hydrogen radical)}$$

$$H_2O \rightarrow H_2O^* \rightarrow H^0 + OH^0 \quad \text{(dissociation)}$$

The free electrons polarize water molecules in the vicinity, forming the relatively long-lived hydrated electron (e_{aq}^-). The hydrated electron and H^0 and OH^0 radicals may diffuse to and react with biomolecules and damage them, so that the cell does not reproduce.

For high-Let radiation, such as recoil protons from scattering of fast neutrons on hydrogen nuclei or alpha particles from radioactive decay, the major action is direct ionization of chemical bonds in the biomolecules. There is also some production of hydrogen peroxide.

Restitution of molecules damaged by indirect action can be achieved, such as by the addition of a free electron:

$$MH^+ + e^- \rightarrow MH$$

or reaction with a hydrogen atom:

$$M^0 + H^0 \rightarrow MH,$$

where M stands for the biomolecule (less H in this example). However, restitution is inhibited by molecular oxygen, which scavenges electrons by

$$O_2 + e^-_{aq} \rightarrow O_2^-$$

and removes organic radicals by peroxydation:

$$M^0 + O_2 \rightarrow MO_2^0$$

Thus, for low-LET (sparsely ionizing) radiation, where indirect action predominates, damage is potentiated by the presence of molecular oxygen. The increase in sensitivity to radiation dose is expressed in terms of the oxygen enhancement ratio (OER):

$$OER = \frac{\text{absorbed dose without oxygen for given effect}}{\text{absorbed dose with oxygen for same effect}} . \qquad (6.21)$$

OER is plotted in Fig. 6.29.

For high-LET (densely ionizing) radiation, such as recoil protons from fast neutron scattering, action is mostly direct and oxygen has little effect.

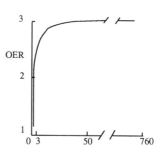

FIG. 6.29 Oxygen enhancement ratio.   Oxygen pressure (mmHg)

In addition to the absorbed dose, it may be useful to define an effective absorbed dose that takes into account LET and any other influences:

$$H = D(\text{RBE}), \tag{6.22}$$

where H is the effective absorbed dose and RBE is the relative biological effectiveness. The unit of effective absorbed dose is the Sievert (Sv), formerly rem when D is given in rad.

$$\text{RBE} = \frac{\text{absorbed dose of 250 kVP x-rays for given effect}}{\text{absorbed dose of radiation for same effect}} . \tag{6.23}$$

RBE depends on the specific biological effect of interest, the type and energy of the ionizing radiation, and the oxygenation of the tissue. In radiobiology, the usual effect is the lethal dose-50 percent (LD50), the absorbed dose required to kill 50 percent of a population of animals, usually within 30 days. In radiotherapy, the effect of interest is the killing of enough malignant cells in a tumor that the body can cope with any viable cells remaining, and so the tumor does not regrow.

The RBE for electrons, gamma rays, and high-energy x-rays is usually the same as for 250 kVp x-rays, hence RBE = 1, assuming normal oxygenation of tissue. For energetic recoil protons, RBE may be 1 to 10. A reduction in molecular oxygen concentration has little if any effect on RBE for high-LET radiation. However, for low-LET radiation, OER (hence RBE) is decreased at low oxygen concentration. This can be a problem, as blood vessels may be damaged during a treatment and the oxygen concentration at the malignant cells may be decreased, thus "protecting" the malignant cells from more damage. The phenomenon of the hypoxic tumor region has lead to interest in applying fast neutrons to radiotherapy, because RBE is not affected by oxygen.

6.8 FRACTIONATION

The reproductive death of malignant cells and other cells is expressed in a cell survival curve, such as shown in Fig. B.1. Such curves can be derived from cell culture experiments in which a colony of reproducing cells grows to visible size from a single viable cell. Similar experiments may be performed in vivo. Note that for high-LET radiation, the cell survival curve is exponential and thus plots as a straight line in log (fraction surviving) versus absorbed dose. For low-LET radiation, however, the semilog plot displays a region of little effect, or shoulder, at low doses. This is explained by repair of sublethal damage, or as a requirement for multiple ionizations in a small volume before enough total damage is done to prevent the cell from reproducing.

To reduce side effects from radiotherapy, it is standard practice in radio-

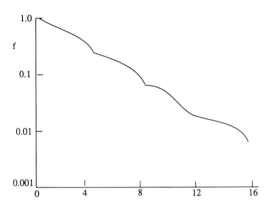

FIG. 6.30   Surviving fraction f vs. dose (gray). Fractionated treatment.

therapy with low-LET radiation to distribute the absorbed dose over several fractions as shown in Fig. 6.30. For example, the radiotherapist may prescribe 2 to 4 Gy per day until some 40 to 60 Gy is accumulated at the tumor. Because the absorbed dose at the beginning of each irradiation has little effect, the total absorbed dose has to be increased. However, reoxygenation of the tumor may occur by delivering the dose in fractions. Furthermore, advantage may be taken of cell reproduction kinetics and radiosensitivity of nonmalignant cells, so that fractionating the absorbed dose favors partial recovery of the nonmalignant tissue between irradiations.

BIBLIOGRAPHY

Bushong, S. C. 1988. *Radiologic science for Technologists*. 4th ed. St. Louis: C. V. Mosby.

Cameron, J. R., and J. G. Skofronick. 1978. *Medical physics*, Chap. 16. New York: John Wiley & Sons.

Hall, E. J. 1978. *Radiobiology for the radiologist*. 2d ed. Hagerstown, Md.: Harper & Row.

Hendee, W. R. 1979. *Medical radiation physics*. 2d ed. Chicago: Year Book Medical Publishers.

Hubbell, J. H. 1969. *Photon cross sections, attenuation coefficients, and energy absorption coefficients from 10 keV to 100 GeV*. NRDS-NBS 29. Washington: U.S. Government Printing Office.

Knoll, G. F. 1989. *Radiation detection and measurement*. 2d ed. New York: John Wiley & Sons.

Profio, A. E. 1979. *Radiation shielding and dosimetry*, New York: John Wiley & Sons.

Robb, R. A. 1982. X-ray computed tomography: an engineering synthesis of multi-scientific principles. *CRC Critical Reviews in Biomedical Engineering* Vol. 7(4), (March 1982): 265–333.

Wolfe, J. N. 1972. *Xeroradiography of the breast*. Springfield, Ill.: Charles Thomas.

CHAPTER 7

NUCLEAR MEDICINE

7.1 PRINCIPLES OF NUCLEAR MEDICINE

Nuclear medicine is concerned with measurements using a radioactive form of a drug (radiopharmaceutical) or another radioactive tracer compound. Measurements in vivo usually involve imaging the spatial distribution of the radioisotope in an organ by detection of the emitted gamma rays. The image may be a projected view or a tomographic view. The latter mode is called positron emission tomography (PET) because the energetic photons resulting from the annihilation of positrons are detected. A different kind of tomographic imaging, single photon emission computed tomography (SPECT) uses collimators to define the directions required in CT. Gamma rays (energetic photons of electromagnetic radiation emitted in nuclear-energy–state transitions) are used because they penetrate tissues with relatively little attenuation, and because they deposit only a small fraction of their energy in the tissue (small radiation dose).

For a few tests, most of which involve thyroid function as revealed by the uptake of iodine, a nonimaging detector is sufficient. Then only the total number of detected gamma rays is needed, not the spatial distribution. However, the thyroid might still be imaged to locate benign or malignant tumors, which do not accumulate iodine compound.

A radioactive form of an element behaves chemically the same as a stable form. It is also possible to "tag" a compound with a few radioactive atoms, even if these atoms are not found in the natural form of the compound. Thus, an important advantage of nuclear medicine as compared with x-ray transmission (diagnostic radiology) is its ability to reveal physiology as well as anatomy. If an image is accumulated rapidly, the time dependence of the uptake and distribution can be studied, that is, the pharmacokinetics and pharmacodynamics.

Many tests (for example, tests on blood serum) are now made in vitro using radioisotope-labeled reagents. The radioisotope may be a beta particle. Beta particles are energetic electrons emitted in some nuclear transformations, especially in radioactive decay. They have a small range in solids or liquids (on the order of millimeters). However, they can be detected in a thin film. Even very low-energy beta particles can be detected if the labeled compound is mixed with a liquid organic scintillator.

7.2 RADIOACTIVITY AND RADIONUCLIDES

A nuclide is designated by ^{A}S, where S is the chemical symbol of the element and A is the nucleon number, the sum of the number of protons and the number of neutrons in the nucleus. The number of protons is Z, the atomic number, which may be derived from the chemical symbol. Isotopes are nuclides of the same Z but different A. Isomers are pairs of nuclides, one in an metastable excited-state, ^{Am}S and the other ground state ^{A}S. Usually, the terms *isotope* and *radioisotope* are used for stable and radioactive species, respectively.

Modes of Decay

Radioactivity is a process in which an unstable nucleus transforms (decays) into a stable or less unstable nucleus, with emission of particles or gamma rays. Modes of radioactive decay are listed in Table 7.1.

Alpha decay (emission of an α particle or nucleus of ^{4}He), spontaneous fission, and internal conversion (conversion of gamma ray energy to an electron) are of no importance in nuclear medicine. This leaves negatron beta decay (emission of a broad spectrum of electrons, from 0 to a couple MeV), positron beta decay (emission of a broad spectrum of positrons), electron capture, and isomeric transition as the principal modes of radioactive decay used in nuclear medicine. Gamma rays are often emitted immediately fol-

TABLE 7.1 Radioactive Decay Modes

Mode	Product Nucleus	Radiations (Spectrum)
Alpha	Z − 2, A − 4	α (line), often γ (line)
Negatron beta	Z + 1, A	β − (continuous), often γ
Positron beta	Z − 1, A	β + (continuous), often γ
Electron capture (EC)	Z − 1, A	X or Auger e −
Internal conversion (IC)	Z, A	e$^-$ (line)
Isomeric transition (IT)	Z, A	γ (line)
Spontaneous fission	Z/2, A/2 (approx.)	n, γ (continuous)

lowing beta decay. In positron beta decay, two annihilation quanta are emitted, each of 551 keV energy and 180° to each other, when the positron combines with an electron. In electron capture, an orbital electron (usually K-shell) is absorbed by the nucleus, leaving a vacancy soon filled by outer electrons, with emission of x-rays or low-energy (Auger) electrons. Isomeric transition involves emission of a monoenergetic gamma ray corresponding to the transition between a metastable excited state and the ground, or minimum energy, state of a nucleus.

Activity and Half-Life

The number of transformations per unit time (decays/sec) is called the *activity*. The number of gamma rays of a certain energy emitted per unit time is equal to the activity multiplied by the fraction of transformations that result in emission of the gamma ray of that energy (not necessarily 100 percent, because of competition by other modes of decay or branching to another energy level, hence a different emitted gamma ray energy). The SI unit of activity is the becquerel (Bq), where

$$1 \text{ Bq} = 1 \text{ transformation/second.} \tag{7.1a}$$

The older unit is the curie (Ci):

$$1 \text{ Ci} = 3.7 \times 10^{10} \text{ transformations/second.} \tag{7.1b}$$

The activity decreases with time because of the transformations into a more stable state. At any instant,

$$A = \lambda N, \tag{7.2}$$

where λ is the decay constant and N is the number of radioactive nuclei at that instant. The rate of decrease in N is equal to the activity, hence

$$dN/dt = -\lambda N \tag{7.3}$$

and the activity at any time is

$$A(t) = A_0 \exp(-\lambda t), \tag{7.4}$$

where A_0 is the activity at $t = 0$. Instead of the decay constant, it is standard practice to give the half-life T, the duration for the activity to equal half of the activity at the beginning of the time interval,

$$A(T) = 0.5A_0. \tag{7.5}$$

It follows that

$$T = \ln 2/\lambda = 0.693/\lambda. \tag{7.6}$$

Radionuclides

A list of radionuclides commonly used in nuclear medicine is given in Table 7.2. The mode of decay, energy of any gamma rays emitted, maximum energy of any beta particles emitted, and half-life are listed. The table lists radionuclides that emit gamma rays, those that emit positrons (hence, also annihilation quanta), and those that emit only negatron beta particles (no gamma rays).

Production

Probably the most widely used radionuclide is ^{99m}Tc. It is obtained as sodium pertechnate ($Na^{99m}TcO_4$) by elution with saline from a ^{99}Mo-^{99m}Tc radionuclide generator such as shown in Fig. 7.1. Although the half-life of ^{99m}Tc is only 6 h, it is the daughter of 67 h ^{99}Mo, which is produced by neutron

TABLE 7.2 Radioisotopes Used in Nuclear Medicine

Nuclide	Mode	Gamma Energy keV (frac.)	Beta Energy keV	Half-Life
^{51}Cr	EC	320 (10%)	—	27.7 d
^{67}Ga	EC	92	—	78.3 h
^{81m}Kr	IT	190	0	13 s[1]
^{99m}Tc	IT	140	0	6 h[2]
^{111}In	EC	387	—	67.4 h
^{123}I	EC	160 (84%)	—	13 h
^{131}I	β−	364 (88%)	192	8.1 d
^{133}Xe	β−	81	346	5.3 d
^{201}Tl	EC	167 (12%)	—	73 h
^{11}C	β+	511 (200%)	961	20.4 m
^{13}N	β+	511 (200%)	1190	10.0 m
^{15}O	β+	511 (200%)	1723	122 s
^{18}F	β+	511 (200%)	635	110 m
^{3}H	β−	0	18.6	12.3 y
^{14}C	β−	0	155	5730 y

[1]Daughter of 4.6 hours ^{81}Rb.
[2]Daughter of 66 hours ^{99}Mo.

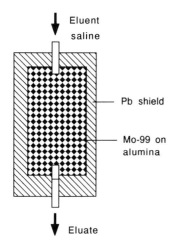

Eluent saline

Pb shield

Mo-99 on alumina

Eluate

Tc-99m (pertechnate) **FIG. 7.1** Mo-99/Tc-99m generator.

capture in molydenum in a nuclear reactor. The ^{99m}Tc comes into equilibrium with the ^{99}Mo and decays at the same rate as the parent, and thus ^{99m}Tc is readily available. The pertechnate is reduced to ionic technetium (with stannous chloride), then complexed with the desired compound. The necessary sterile, pyrogen-free chemicals come as a kit, lyophilized and under an inert gas. Then the sodium pertechnate is added just before use, and the labeled compound is ready for use in a few minutes. The labeling efficiency (the activity in the labeled compound as compared with total activity) may be 90 to 99 percent. A radionuclide generator is also used for preparation of the short-lived ^{81m}Kr from the longer-lived ^{81}Rb. Negatron beta-emitting radionuclides are usually produced by neutron irradiation in a nuclear reactor. Their half-lives are long enough to permit preparation elsewhere. ^{131}I is a fission product.

The positron-emitting radioisotopes of abundant elements in the body (C, N, O, and F as an analog of H) have very short half-lives and must be produced near the point of use. These radionuclides are made by bombardment of a target with charged particles (p, d, or α) in a cyclotron. Radionuclides decaying by electron capture are also prepared by charged-particle bombardment, but have half-lives long enough for them to be produced elsewhere and shipped when needed.

7.3 RADIOPHARMACEUTICALS

A radionuclide-tagged compound must be radiochemically and chemically pure, sterile, and nonpyrogenic if injected. Most radiopharmaceuticals are injected intravenously, but thyroid uptake of radioiodine is usually studied by the patient's swallowing a solution of sodium iodide. Once in the blood, the radiopharmaceutical is circulated and may accumulate preferentially in certain tissues, e.g., malignant tumors. The drug may be metabolized and the metabolites eliminated in the urine or feces. Some mechanisms for localization of radiopharmaceuticals are summarized in Table 7.3 along with examples.

A radionuclide should be taken up in greater (or lesser) concentration in the organ or tumor to be examined than in normal surrounding tissue. Moreover, the radionuclide should be cleared rapidly from blood, where it only adds to background and reduces contrast. Sometimes the removal of a radionuclide is exponential, with a "biological decay constant" (λ_b) or a "biological half-life" (T_b). If the radioactive decay constant is λ_d (or the half-life for radioactive decay is T_d), the combined decay constant and half-life for the exponential reduction in activity in a certain organ are as follows:

$$\lambda_t = \lambda_b + \lambda_d \tag{7.7}$$

$$1/T_t = 1/T_b + 1/T_d. \tag{7.8}$$

Technetium-99m

The pertechnate ($^{99m}TcO_4^-$) may be administered orally or intravenously and behaves in the body like iodine. It concentrates in the thyroid, salivary glands, stomach, and choroid plexus. About 50 percent is diluted from blood plasma into the extravascular space in 15 to 20 minutes. The remaining activity disappears from plasma with a half-life of some 3 hours. About 20 to 30 percent of the activity is eventually eliminated in the feces. Presumably the rest decays or may be eliminated in urine. Some 20 percent of the activity remains in stomach for several hours. Pertechnate is currently the radiopharmaceutical of choice for brain scanning and is also used for scanning the thyroid, salivary glands, and stomach.

TABLE 7.3 Mechanisms for Localization of Radiopharmaceuticals

Method	Example
Active transport	Thyroid uptake and scanning with I
Compartmental localization	Blood pool scanning with human serum albumin, plasma, or RBC volume
Simple exchange or diffusion	Bone scanning with ^{99m}Tc-phosphate
Phagocytosis	Liver, spleen, and bone marrow scans with radiocolloid
Capillary blockade	Lung scanning and organ perfusion scans with labeled macroaggregates
Cell sequestration	Spleen scan with damaged RBCs.

^{99m}Tc-labeled sulfur colloid is removed from blood by reticuloendothelial cells. The distribution among the organs with reticuloendothelial cells depends on the size and the type of the colloidal particles, the blood supply, and other physiological conditions. For sulfur colloid with a particle size of about 0.3 μm, 70 to 80 percent is localized in the liver within 10 to 20 minutes of intravenous injection. About 15 to 20 percent is localized in bone marrow and 3 percent in the spleen. Thus ^{99m}Tc-labeled sulfur colloid is used to scan these organs.

^{99m}Tc-labeled macroaggregated albumin (MAA), with particle sizes between 15 and 75 μm, is used primarily for lung scanning. In a few seconds after intravenous injection, some 90 to 95 percent of the labeled MAA is trapped in capillary and precapillary beds of the lung. Perfusion of the lung with blood can be studied.

^{99m}Tc-labeled polyphosphate, pyrophosphate, and diphosphonate are used mostly for bone scanning. Some 50 to 60 percent of the activity is localized in the skeleton in 15 to 20 minutes after intravenous injection. The rest is distributed in soft tissue and plasma and excreted slowly in urine. About 20 to 30 percent of the activity is either excreted or taken up by the kidneys within 3 hours of injection. Methylene diphosphonate (MDP) has the fastest rate of plasma clearance and is therefore preferred. However, ^{99m}Tc pyrophosphate and diphosphonate are useful for detection of myocardial infarctions.

^{99m}Tc-labeled red blood cells (RBCs) may be prepared by first coating the RBCs with stannous chloride (injecting an unlabeled pyrophosphate solution) and then, after minutes, injecting the pertechnate. The RBCs can be damaged by heating them in a water bath to 50° C for 30 minutes. Damaged RBCs may be used for scanning the spleen.

^{99m}Tc-labeled 2,3-dimercapto succinic acid (DMSA) is the radiopharmaceutical of choice for studying the morphology of the renal cortex. The biological half-life in the plasma, after intravenous injection, is about 1 hour. At 2 hours, 40 to 50 percent of the injected activity is in the renal cortex and about 15 percent is excreted in the urine. This radiopharmaceutical decomposes rapidly and should be prepared just before use and stored in a refrigerator if necessary.

^{99m}Tc-labeled diethyltriamine pentaacetic acid (DTPA) is used for brain and kidney scanning. The biological half-life in plasma is about 15 minutes. About 80 percent of the injected activity appears in the urine between 2 and 3 hours after injection. Another compound for brain and kidney scanning is ^{99m}Tc-labeled glucoheptonate, which may also be used for detection of myocardial infarction.

^{99m}Tc-labeled HIDA, Diethyl-IDA, PIPIDA, and DISIDA have displaced ^{131}I-labeled rose bengal for imaging the hepatobiliary system. ^{99m}Tc HIDA is rapidly cleared from the blood by hepatocytes, with a biological half-life of several minutes. The compound is rapidly transferred to the bile and thence to the intestine. More than 70 percent of the injected activity appears in the intestine within an hour, and 15 percent in the urine. The transport and excretion of these compounds depend on the patency of the system, e.g., the gallbladder and duct.

Radioiodine

^{131}I is being replaced by ^{123}I because the radiation dose is smaller. Iodine-131 is still used sometimes because of its low cost and freedom from other radioisotopes of iodine. Iodine is generally administered orally because it is readily absorbed by the stomach. After intravenous administration (or when orally administered, after absorption in blood), iodide ion is distributed throughout extracellular water. Then it is slowly taken up by thyroid, stomach, intestine, salivary gland, and choroid plexus. A large fraction is excreted in urine by the kidneys. By 24 hours, 75 percent of the activity is excreted, 15 percent is taken up by the thyroid to form thyroid hormones, 4 to 5 percent is in the gastrointestinal (GI) tract, and 1 to 2 percent circulates in the blood. In hyperthyroidism, the disease characterized by excessive production of thyroid hormones, the thyroid may take up 90 percent of the radioiodine with almost no excretion. In hypothyroidism, in which there is too little production of thyroid hormones, only 1 to 2 percent of the radioactive iodide may be taken up by the thyroid, and 95 percent excreted. Radioiodine is widely used to measure thyroid function and to image the thyroid.

^{123}I-hippuran is rapidly cleared by the kidneys and is used to study the time dependence of renal function. ^{123}I-isopropylamphetamine and similar drugs are used for measuring brain function, especially regional blood flow.

Other Radiopharmaceuticals

^{67}Ga citrate is employed in the diagnosis of soft-tissue tumors and inflammatory diseases. After intravenous administration, about 30 percent of the activity in blood is bound to plasma proteins, especially transferrin. The remaining gallium diffuses into extracellular space and is slowly cleared by the kidneys to the urine. Some is also excreted in feces. By 24 hours, 15 percent of the activity is in urine, 10 percent in blood, and the rest in kidney, bone, liver, and lymph nodes. The biological half-life of gallium is 1 to 2 weeks.

^{51}Cr-labeled RBCs are used to determine the RBC volume and mean life. The patient's own RBCs are used. Blood is withdrawn and incubated with acid dextrose and sodium chromate-151, ascorbic acid is added, and the mixture is reinjected into the patient. ^{51}Cr^{+++} not bound to cells is excreted in urine.

^{201}Tl as thallous chloride is of interest for detection of myocardial infarction and ischemia. Thallium behaves in the body like potassium, which is localized intracellularly. After intravenous injection, it is cleared from blood with a biological half-life of 4 minutes, and, except in the brain (no absorption), it is localized more or less in proportion to the blood supply. At 15 to 20 minutes after injection, 4 percent of the activity is in the myocardium, 12 percent in the liver, 4 percent in the kidneys, and most of the rest in body muscles. The biological half-life for removal of thallous ions from the organs is about 10 days. There is reduced uptake of thallous ion in the myocardium if the blood supply is impaired (ischemia), or if the cells are damaged (infarction).

^{111}In-labeled DPTA is the radiopharmaceutical of choice for imaging the cerebrospinal fluid (CSF). When injected intrathecally, it rises to the basal cisterns in 2 to 3 hours. By 24 to 48 hours, the activity rises over convexities of the brain and into the parasagittal area. Then it is reabsorbed into the blood and quickly excreted by the kidneys into urine. ^{111}In-labeled platelets are used for thrombus detection. ^{111}In-labeled leukocytes are used for abscess detection. However, the difficulty of labeling platelets or leukocytes prevents widespread adoption of this agent. ^{111}In-labeled monoclonal antibodies may prove useful for diagnosis of primary tumors and metastases.

^{133}Xe is often used as the gas employed to study lung ventilation. Dissolved in saline and injected, it may be used for studies of lung perfusion and blood flow. The biological half-life of ^{133}Xe is only a few minutes. Some 2 percent may be held by fat, however, with a biological half-life of about 10 hours. Xenon-133 may be replaced by ^{81m}Kr because its short half-life allows repeated measurements to be made within a few minutes.

^{3}H and ^{14}C are pure beta emitters with very low energies. They are mostly useful in labeling organic compounds when such a compound can be detected by liquid scintillation counting, or in a thin film (such as a chromatogram). Imaging of very thin tissue specimens can be performed by the technique of autoradiography, in which a labeled specimen is placed in intimate contact with a nuclear emulsion (a thick, high-grain–density photographic emulsion). After days or weeks, the emulsion is processed like photographic film and the image examined under a microscope.

Positron Emitters

The positron-emitting radionuclides ^{11}C, ^{13}N, ^{15}O, and ^{18}F may be used to label almost any organic compound, including those of physiological interest.

The regional metabolic rate for oxygen (regional oxygen utilization) can be studied by steady-state inhalation of ^{15}O$_2$. The hemoglobin becomes labeled with ^{15}O. Energy from oxidation of organic substances is used to produce adenosine triphosphate (ATP), and the metabolic water generated is labeled with ^{15}O and can be detected. Regional blood flow can be measured by the inhalation of C^{15}O$_2$. The oxygen-15 label is rapidly and completely transferred to the water pool of the alveolar lung tissue, thus labeling circulating water. The distribution of the water depends on the blood flow to the various regions of the body. Other radiopharmaceuticals for measuring regional blood flow include ^{13}NH$_3$, ^{13}N$_2$O, and a number of ^{11}C-labeled compounds such as methane, acetylene, iodoantipyrine, and ^{11}C-labeled microspheres. A particularly interesting application is the measurement of regional (e.g., brain) glucose metabolic rate with (^{18}F)-fluoro-2-deoxy-D-glucose (FDG). This is an analog of glucose, which, after phosphorylation, is not metabolized further. FDG is carrier-transported from plasma to the unphosphorylated precursor pool. It can then be transported back to plasma or phosphorylated by an enzyme to FDG-6-PO$_4$.

7.4 DETECTORS

Counters

The standard counter for gamma rays is the thallium-activated sodium iodide scintillation detector, with a lead collimator and shield to define the volume contributing to the counts and to reduce background. The NaI(Tl) crystal may be about 5 cm in diameter by 5 cm thick. An open, or flat-field, collimator is shown in Fig. 7.2. The so-called focused collimator collects gamma rays mainly from a "focal" region. Counts (pulses corresponding to gamma ray interactions) are amplified, a range of pulse heights is selected with a single channel analyzer, and the counts are accumulated in an electronic counter, or "scaler," for a preset time. Alternatively, the average count rate may be obtained and recorded on a strip chart recorder. Gamma ray counters (non-imaging detectors) are often used to diagnose thyroid and kidney function. A typical system for making a renogram is shown in Fig. 7.3.

Anger Camera

The standard imaging device (camera) for gamma ray scintigraphy is the Anger camera. It consists of a collimator, a disc-shaped NaI(Tl) crystal behind the collimator, an array of photomultiplier tubes on the back surface that collects scintillation light, and electronics to derive the position of the scin-

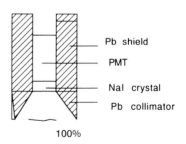

FIG. 7.2 Scintillation detector with open, or flat-field, collimator.

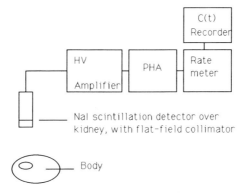

FIG. 7.3 Setup for making a renogram (countrate vs. time).

tillation flash in the crystal as well as the energy from the total amount of light. The physical arrangement is shown in Fig. 7.4. Various collimators are used, depending on the size of the organ to be imaged, the depth, and the spatial resolution. Two Anger cameras are used in SPECT (see Fig. 7.5). The collimator material between holes is thick enough to provide sufficient attenuation for the gamma rays while not reducing efficiency or spatial resolution too much. The NaI(Tl) crystal is typically 1 cm thick and 28 to 45 cm in diameter. The thickness is a compromise between efficiency versus gamma ray energy, and light diffusion. The diameter is large enough to image an entire organ.

The 28-cm disc is fitted with 19 photomultiplier tubes, each 5 cm in di-

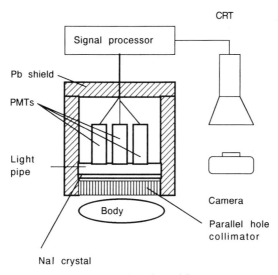

FIG. 7.4 Gamma ray imaging with Anger camera.

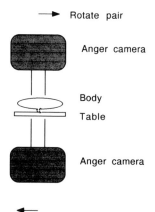

Rotate pair

Anger camera

Body

Table

Anger camera

FIG. 7.5 SPECT arrangement. A pair of Anger cameras is rotated in degree increments about the axis of the body.

ameter. Figure 7.6 shows the principle of light collection for 5 photomultiplier tubes. The light collected by each tube is proportional to the solid angle subtended by the photocathode at the point of the scintillation flash. Figure 7.7 indicates how a circuit can be designed to derive the position coordinates X, Y from the signals from several tubes, X^-, X^+, Y^-, and Y^+. The total signal is Z. Then, for 5 photomultiplier tubes (PMTs),

$$Z = X^+ + X^- + Y^+ + Y^- \tag{7.9a}$$

$$X = K(X^+ - X^-)/Z \tag{7.9b}$$

$$Y = K(Y^+ - Y^-)/Z, \tag{7.9c}$$

where K is a constant.

PET Camera

Positron emission tomography (PET) is similar to x-ray transmission computed tomography (CT), except that the spatial distribution of a radionuclide is measured instead of the attenuation coefficients for x-rays. In both methods, a map of a transverse layer of the body is obtained from measurements with an array of detectors outside the body, based on projections and a computer algorithm. In CT, a measurement of the count rate is made for x-rays traveling along a straight line from the external source to the external detector. In PET, a measurement of count rate is made for gamma rays (annihilation quanta) traveling along a straight line between two external detectors. The basic counter arrangement for PET is shown in Fig. 7.8. The line between counters is defined by the counter dimensions and the requirement for time coincidence. The positron is reduced to low energy and annihilated after traveling a couple of millimeters in tissue. Two annihilation quanta, each of

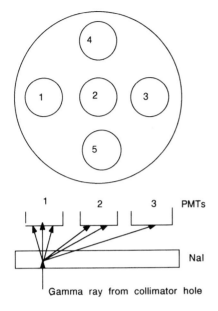

FIG. 7.6 Light division in an Anger camera.

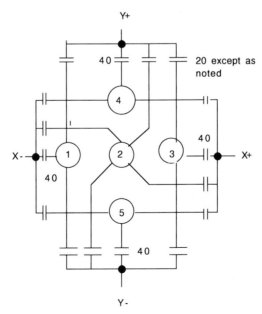

FIG. 7.7 Derivation of position coordinates from PMT signal amplitudes in Anger camera.

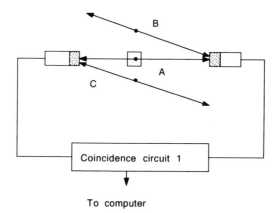

To computer

FIG. 7.8   Principle of a PET system. Annihilation quanta are back-to-back. Coincidence occurs in emission *A*. No coincidence occurs in emission *B*. If emissions occur simultaneously, an accidental coincidence may occur, e.g., between *A* and *C*.

511 keV energy, are emitted back-to-back. Aside from the transit time, they arrive at the two detectors simultaneously. Annihilation quanta not originating on the line are detected by only one counter and are not recorded. At high activities and count rates, however, one quantum in each counter may be detected accidentally within the resolving time interval of the detector and coincidence circuit. These random coincidences are a source of background.

In practice, an array of counters is used, now usually arranged as a ring encircling the body, as seen in Fig. 7.9. The scintillation counters are usually bismuth germanate (BGO), for small size combined with high efficiency at 511 keV. Each counter is placed in time coincidence with many other detectors, so that each pixel in the body is intersected by many lines corresponding to many projections. The same kinds of unfolding algorithms devised for CT can be applied to PET. A correction is made for attenuation of the quanta in tissue. The attenuation factor is the same for one 511 keV photon traversing the entire thickness of the body as for both quanta, each to its own detector. Thus the attenuation factor can be measured by placing a ring of positron

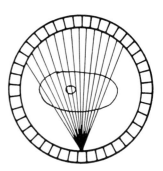

FIG. 7.9   Detector array for a PET scanner.

emitter around the body and measuring the attenuation of one quantum through the body.

Examples of PET images may be seen in Fig. 7.10.

SPECT

Single photon emission computed tomography (SPECT) can use any gamma ray emitter, and thus is not limited to the short-lived positron emitters as is PET. Instead of defining time coincidence, a collimator is used to define the line along which the gamma ray emission is to be measured. SPECT usually

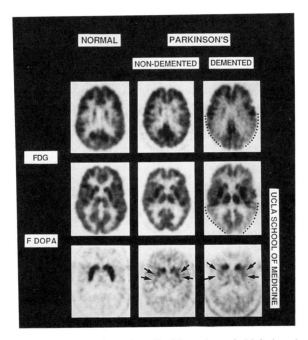

FIG. 7.10 PET images to differentiate Parkinson's and Alzheimer's disease. *Left column*: PET images of glucose metabolism using [18F]-fluorodeoxyglucose (FDG) at high level (*top*) and mid-level of the brain showing the normal pattern. The top and left side of the images are the front and left of the brain. The bottom image shows the pattern of normal dopamine synthesis at the mid-level of the brain as determined with [18F] L-DOPA. The majority of dopamine synthesis is in the central structures of the brain (caudate and putamen). *Center column*: Bottom image shows severe dopamine deficiency of Parkinson's disease, involving primarily the putamen (*arrows*). Glucose metabolism in the upper images is normal. *Right column*: Bottom image shows a dopamine deficiency (*arrows*) consistent with Parkinson's disease. The glucose metabolic images (*top, middle*) show, in addition, that the patient also has the characteristic metabolic deficiency, bilaterally in the parietal and superior temporal cortex (*dotted lines*), of Alzheimer's disease, consistent with the patient's dementia. (Courtesy of S. Grafton, M. Phelps, and J. Mazziotta, UCLA School of Medicine.)

involves one or two Anger cameras mounted on a mechanism that rotates the camera 360° around the patient, stopping to accumulate data at 32 or 64 projection angles. Because the gamma cameras measure the emission over a large area, SPECT can map multiple layers instead of only one. However, differences in tissue attenuation, the variable efficiency of collimation with depth, irregularities in camera sensitivity, and misalignment of rotation affect SPECT adversely. A correction matrix accounting for tissue attenuation may be constructed by rotating through 360° and modeling the body contour. Divergence of the collimator and counts from Compton scattered gamma rays may be reduced by making a special collimator with a smaller acceptance angle. The same computer unfolding algorithms can be used for SPECT as for PET and CT.

7.5   COUNTING STATISTICS AND BACKGROUND

The images accumulated in nuclear medicine, like all nuclear measurements, are subject to statistical variations. Radioactive decay is a random process: it is not possible to tell when a certain nucleus will decay, only the probability of decay for a large number of radioactive nuclei. The emission of gamma rays or other radiations follows the same statistical variation. In nuclear medicine, one may speak of counts (detected events) or counts per unit area of the image. These counts are accumulated over a certain time interval. The objective is to administer sufficient activity in a radiopharmaceutical so that the number of counts accumulated over the available duration of the measurement is great enough that the statistical variation is small.

The distribution of the number of counts equal to N, when the mean number of counts is M, is given by the Poisson distribution for the probability P:

$$P(N) = M^N e^{-M}/N! \tag{7.10}$$

The Poisson distribution, for $N > 20$, is very close to the normal distribution with a standard deviation of

$$\sigma = M^{0.5}. \tag{7.11}$$

The best estimate of the true mean M is the average of a series of measurements. In nuclear medicine imaging, usually only one measurement (image) is made, and this has to be taken as the mean. The standard deviation is the square root of the mean. Thus, if a pixel contains, for example, 100 counts, the standard deviation is 10 counts. Another image might give 90 to 110 counts or even greater deviation. That is, for a mean of 100 counts, 68 percent of the measurements should lie within plus or minus 10, one standard deviation. The fractional standard deviation σ/M is 10 percent. For 1000 counts, the estimated standard deviation is 31.6 counts (3.2 percent), and for 10,000 counts the fractional standard deviation is 1 percent. If the standard deviation is larger than the difference of activity, and hence, mean counts in two volumes of tissue, it will not be possible to determine whether there is really a difference in activity in the two volumes or only a statistical fluctuation and image quality will be poor. Because of the very low geometrical efficiency encountered in nuclear medicine, it is quite likely that statistical precision will be poor even for relatively large values of activity per unit volume.

Nuclear measurements, including nuclear medicine imaging, often suffer from a large background that should be minimized and subtracted. For example, in imaging with an Anger camera, gamma rays are contributed by activity in blood and in tissue located above and below the level of interest, or scattered onto the collimator hole. If a way can be found to measure background, the mean counts per pixel from the desired layer can be found by subtracting the mean background. As discussed in section 1.2, the standard deviation of the net counts is equal to the square root of the sum of the squares of the standard deviations of background and background-plus-radioisotope gamma rays.

7.6 RADIATION DOSE

The biological effects of gamma rays and electrons in tissue are correlated with the absorbed dose (energy deposited by ionization and excitation, per unit mass of tissue). Absorbed dose is given in grays (1 Gy = 1 J/kg) or the older unit, rad = 0.01 J/kg. Specialists in nuclear medicine have expended considerable effort in predicting the absorbed dose to various organs, for the radionuclides of interest, per curie or becquerel of activity administered. Experience has also been gained in the activity that must be administered to carry out various nuclear medicine procedures and with the absorbed dose the patient receives from this activity until the radionuclide either decays or is eliminated from the body.

The first step is to make an inventory of the energy (average energy for beta particles) according to the particle, low-energy x-ray, or gamma ray emitted in radioactive decay. This, together with the determination of the activity and fraction going by each pathway, gives the rate of energy released in short-range charged particles (or small mean free-path x-rays) and the rate of energy released in gamma rays of given energy. Usually, the charged particles and low-energy x-rays are assumed to be absorbed where they are released; therefore, the absorbed-dose rate in an organ is equal to the energy-release rate from activity in that organ, for these radiations.

Next, the attenuation coefficient for tissue (or for soft and hard tissues) at the gamma ray energy has to be known, a model constructed for the geometry and mass of the major organs in the body, and a method devised to determine the distribution of gamma rays throughout the body from gamma rays released in a given organ. These calculations are often done on a com-

TABLE 7.4   Radiation Dose in Nuclear Medicine Procedures

Procedure	Activity (mCi)	Dose (rad)	Organ
Brain scan ($^{99m}TcO_4^-$)	10	2–3	stomach
Bone scan (^{99m}Tc phosphate)	10	1–2	bladder
Liver scan (^{99m}Tc S colloid)	3	1	liver
Lung scan (^{133}Xe)	10	0.3	lung
Thyroid scan (^{123}I)	0.1	1.5–3.0	thyroid
(^{131}I)	0.05	60–90	thyroid
Spleen (^{51}Cr damaged RBCs)	0.25	5–12	spleen
Kidney (^{99m}Tc DTPA)	20	2–5	bladder
Heart (^{201}Tl chloride)	1.5	2.2	kidneys
Liver-gallbladder (^{99m}Tc HIDA)	5	1.6	sm. intestine
Cisternography (^{111}In DPTA)	0.5	1.9	spinal cord
Tumor (^{67}Ga citrate)	5	4.5	colon

puter by the Monte Carlo radiation transport method. The calculation also yields the energy absorbed from the gamma ray, given the energy absorption coefficient for the tissue (which depends on gamma ray energy). The result is the absorbed fraction, $\phi(T \leftarrow S)$, which is defined as the amount of energy absorbed in a target volume, T, divided by the amount of energy emitted in source volume S. If the target is the same as the source volume, this becomes the absorbed fraction ϕ, which has been tabulated for various organs and gamma ray energies. The process of dose calculation has been simplified by tabulation of the S factor for a specific radionuclide, which is

$$S = K \sum_i n_i E_i \, \phi_i(T \leftarrow S), \qquad (7.8)$$

n_i is the fraction of decays giving the ith gamma ray, E_i is the energy of the ith gamma ray, $\phi(T \leftarrow S)$ is the ith absorbed fraction and K is a units conversion constant. The factors have been tabulated in the MIRD pamphlets, a supplement to the *Journal of Nuclear Medicine*. Radiopharmaceutical, activity administered, and radiation dose to critical organs are listed for some procedures in Table 7.4.

BIBLIOGRAPHY

Cameron, J. R., and J. G. Skofronick. 1978. *Medical Physics*. New York: John Wiley & Sons, pp. 438–478.

Chandra, R. 1987. *Introductory physics of nuclear medicine*. 3d ed. Philadelphia: Lea & Febiger.

Lammertsma, A. A., and R. S. J. Frackowiak. 1985. Position emission tomography. *CRC Critical Reviews in Biomedical Engineering* 13(2):125–169.

CHAPTER 8

DIAGNOSTIC ULTRASOUND

8.1 PRINCIPLES OF ULTRASOUND

Ultrasound is defined as sound waves with frequencies above the range of human hearing, about 20 kHz. A sound wave consists of zones of alternate compression and rarefaction, generated by a moving surface. The wave is longitudinal, in that it propagates through matter in the same direction as the compression and rarefaction. The speed of sound in the medium (v_s), the wavelength (λ), and the frequency (f) of the wave are related as follows:

$$v_s = f\lambda \tag{8.1}$$

The speed of sound in soft tissues is about 1540 m/s. The wavelength for diagnostic purposes should be on the order of 1 mm or less. Thus the frequency should be on the order of 1.5 MHz or greater. Diagnostic imaging typically uses frequencies between 1 and 15 MHz.

The speed of sound depends on the density and compressibility of the medium. The higher the density and the lower the compressibility, the higher the speed. Thus the speed is low in air, higher in soft tissues, and highest in bone. Speeds are listed in Table 8.1 for some tissues and materials of interest.

Imaging by ultrasound is based on reflection of sound waves at an interface between two media of different acoustic impedance, Z, where

$$Z = \rho v_s. \tag{8.2}$$

TABLE 8.1 Speed and Acoustic Impedance of Biologic Interest

Tissue	v_s (m/s)	$Z \ (kg - m^{-2} - s^{-1}) \times 10^{-4}$
Fat	1475	1.38
Brain	1560	1.55
Liver	1570	1.65
Kidney	1560	1.62
Spleen	1570	1.64
Blood	1570	1.61
Muscle	1570	1.70
Lens of eye	1620	1.85
Skull bone	3360	6.10
Ave. soft tissue	1540	1.63
Water (25°C)	1498	1.50
Air	331	0.0004

Some values for Z are listed in Table 8.1. The fraction of beam energy reflected at an interface is

$$\alpha_r = \left(\frac{Z_2 - Z_1}{Z_2 + Z_1}\right)^2, \tag{8.3}$$

assuming perpendicular incidence. The fraction transmitted is $1 - \alpha_r$. For example, at a muscle-kidney interface, $Z_1 = 1.70 \times 10^{-4}$ and $Z = 1.62 \times 10^{-4}$. Then $\alpha_r = 0.00058$. These considerations apply to specular reflection. If the interface is rough or the medium is very inhomogeneous, diffuse scattering occurs.

If the sound beam is incident on the interface at an angle θ_i to the normal, the transmitted beam is refracted and has an angle to the normal of θ_t. The relationship of the angles is given by Snells's law:

$$\frac{\sin \theta_i}{\sin \theta_t} = \frac{v_s(\text{incidence medium})}{v_s(\text{refractive medium})}. \tag{8.4}$$

If the sound speed increases upon entering the second medium, the wave can be refracted out of the medium, and total internal reflection occurs. Refraction is a source of artifacts in diagnostic imaging.

The intensity of the ultrasound beam is a compromise between the intensity that might cause biologic effects ($100 \ mW/cm^2$ for long exposure to a continuous wave beam) and the intensity required for detection of the reflected sound or "echo" allowing for attenuation and losses upon reflection. Diagnostic ultrasound intensity is typically 1 to 10 mW/cm^2. The sound wave is attenuated by "relaxation" or frictional processes in the medium that convert acoustic energy into heat. The attenuation is exponential. The change in

TABLE 8.2   Attenuation Coefficients for 1 MHz Ultrasound

Tissue	α (dB/cm)
Blood	0.18
Fat	0.6
Muscle (across fibers)	3.3
Muscle (along fibers)	1.2
Eye humors	0.1
Lens of eye	2.0
Skull bone	20.0
Lung	40.0
Liver	0.9
Brain	0.85
Kidney	1.0
Spinal cord	1.0
Water	0.0022

intensity is usually described in terms of the logarithm of the ratio, with units of decibels:

$$\text{Intensity ratio (dB)} = 10 \log \frac{I}{I_o}. \qquad (8.5)$$

Thus attenuation by a factor of 10 would be described as -10 dB. Intensity is proportional to the square of the wave pressure, hence the intensity ratio for pressure is -20 dB in the example. The attenuation coefficient is usually given in terms of dB/cm of tissue thickness traversed. The attenuation coefficient differs widely depending on the particular tissue. Values are listed in Table 8.2. The values are temperature dependent.

8.2 TRANSDUCER AND BEAM

The transducer used to both excite and detect ultrasound waves is a piezo-electric crystal. Applying a voltage across the crystal faces causes mechanical strain (either expansion or compression, depending on the polarity). The crystal is coupled to the medium and excited with an alternating voltage to generate ultrasound waves in the medium. Conversely, ultrasound waves received at the crystal cause strain, which results in a voltage across the crystal. The relationship between strain (S) and electric field intensity (E) is

$$S = \text{change in crystal thickness/original crystal thickness} \qquad (8.6)$$
$$= gE$$

Some values of g are given in Table 8.3, for crystals often used in piezoelectric transducers. The efficiency in converting mechanical energy to electrical energy, or the reverse, is given by the square of the electromechanical coupling coefficient, k_c, also listed in Table 8.3. Finally, the curie point is listed. Above the curie point temperature, piezoelectric properties are lost, and an ultrasound transducer should never be exposed to higher temperatures.

A typical ultrasound transducer is shown in Fig. 8.1. The piezoelectric element (crystal) is circular and located at one end of the case. The thickness of the crystal is either one-half or one-quarter of the wavelength of sound in the crystal, for a mechanical resonance and maximum efficiency in ultrasound generation and reception. A matching layer protects the crystal and, with an acoustic impedance between that of the crystal and tissue, maximizes coupling into the tissue. It is important to exclude air, and a gel may be used between the transducer and the skin to match impedances. The crystal may be planar, or concave for a focusing effect. An acoustic lens may be used to focus the ultrasound. Because the speed of sound is greater in the lens material than in air, focusing is achieved with a concave lens and defocusing is achieved

TABLE 8.3 Properties of Piezoelectric Transducer Crystals

Material	g (m/V) $\times$ 10^{-12}	k_c	Curie pt (°C)
Quartz	2.3	0.11	550
Barium titanate	60–190	0.30	120
Lead zirconate titanate (PET-4)	290	0.70	328
Lead zirconate titanate (PET-5)	370	0.70	365

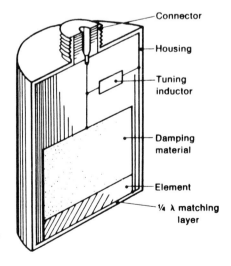

FIG. 8.1 Typical ultrasound transducer. (Courtesy of Dapco Industries, Ridgefield, Conn.)

with a convex lens. The damping material (e.g., tungsten powder in epoxy) suppresses reverberation, so that the crystal stops vibrating soon after the exciting voltage is removed. Damping is not required for Doppler applications, in which a continuous sinusoidal wave is applied.

Most imaging applications use the pulse-echo technique, where the crystal is excited (for example, for 2 to 5 cycles) at the ultrasound frequency, followed by a long time during which reflected sound pulses are received by the same transducer. For instance, at 2.5 MHz, the pulse duration may be 1 μs (2.5 cycles), followed by a quiet period of 999 μs during which reflected pulses arrive. The pulse repetition frequency is 1 kHz. Consider that the round-trip transit time for a 30 cm thick body, at a speed of 1540 m/s, is

$$t = \frac{2d}{v_s}$$

$$= \frac{2(0.3)}{1540} = 390 \ \mu s. \tag{8.7}$$

Equation 8.7 can be used to find the depth of any reflecting interface from the measured time delay, provided the speed of sound is known. There is actually a range of frequencies associated with the sound pulse, because it is short. The range may be expressed as a bandwidth or the quality factor (center frequency divided by bandwidth).

The propagation of an ultrasound beam from a transducer can be visualized in terms of wave fronts. A wave front is a curve tangent to the compression or rarefaction zone. For a large flat transducer, the wave fronts are planar. For a small source, approximating a point, the wave fronts are spherical. The wave fronts for an intermediate-size source can be derived by considering each point on the transducer to be a source of spherical waves. It is necessary to consider interference between waves from different points. When two waves (of equal frequency) are in phase, constructive interference occurs. When the waves are 180° out of phase, destructive interference occurs. The resultant beam is illustrated schematically in Fig. 8.2. The region near the transducer is called the *near-field* or *Fresnel zone*. The region farther from

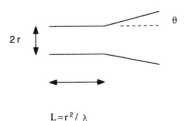

$L = r^2 / \lambda$

FIG. 8.2 Schematic of ultrasound beam with Fresnel and Fraunhofer zones.

the transducer is called the *far-field* or *Fraunhofer zone*. For a disk-shaped transducer of radius r, the length L of the Fresnel zone is

$$L = \frac{r^2}{\lambda} . \tag{8.8}$$

Most of the sound energy is confined to a beam equal to the transducer diameter. This is the region desired for diagnostic ultrasound applications. In the Fraunhofer zone, the beam diverges with a half-angle θ, where

$$\sin \theta = 0.612 \frac{\lambda}{r} . \tag{8.9}$$

For a frequency of 2 MHz and a transducer radius of 1.0 cm, $L = 13.3$ cm and $\theta = 2.6°$.

The beam may also be described in terms of echo amplitude versus axial distance and lateral spread, or by isoecho contours. These have to be measured, e.g., by placing a small reflecting object at various positions. The lateral distribution may be more or less Gaussian, with the width expressed by the -6 dB or -20 dB point, relative to the amplitude on axis. The beam is attenuated in tissue so that the isoecho contour resembles a narrow loop. Small side lobes may be present around the primary beam, which could cause artifacts near the transducer. Another source of artifacts is standing waves, which can exist when incident and reflected waves travel in opposite directions and interfere with each other. They can be eliminated by adjusting the position or the angle of the transducer.

Axial resolution is the ability of two closely spaced reflecting objects on the transducer axis to be distinguished. It is determined by the length of the pulse. If the pulse includes 2 to 5 cycles, the axial resolution will be 2 to 5 wavelengths. Higher frequency improves the axial resolution. Lateral resolution is the ability of two closely spaced objects in a plane perpendicular to the axis to be distinguished. It is determined by the diameter of the transducer (large diameter gives poorer resolution) and by the frequency (higher frequency gives better resolution). Lateral resolution is very important in diagnostic imaging applications. A typical scan of the abdomen at 2.5 MHz may have an axial resolution of 2 mm, but a lateral resolution of only 1 to 2 cm. For examination of the lens of the eye, in which great depth of penetration is not required, the frequency can be 10 MHz and the lateral resolution some 2 mm.

Several transducer crystals may be mounted together to form a linear transducer array, such as illustrated in Fig. 8.3. For example, 32 rectangular crystals each 2 mm wide may be mounted in an array 6.4 cm long. Only 1 crystal is excited and receiving at one time. The crystals can be excited in sequence from 1 to 32, giving 32 scan lines in the frame. Arrays are often excited segmentally, with 5 contiguous crystals energized at once, giving 5

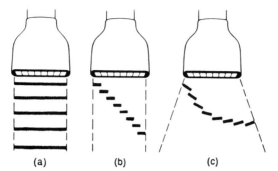

FIG. 8.3 Transducer array and wave fronts. (From Bushong, S. C. 1988. *Radiologic science for technologists*. 4th ed. St. Louis: C. V. Mosby.)

scan lines. For example, crystals 1 through 5 may be energized in one pulse, then crystals 2 through 6 in another pulse, and so on. If a delay is then introduced between excitation of each crystal, the transducer becomes a phased array and the beam can approximate a sector scan (up to 90°). The scan lines can be 1 mm apart and the sector scan can have 1° between scan lines; however, the lateral resolution would be much poorer. The advantage of the phased array is that a real-time image can be seen without moving the transducer.

In pulse-echo imaging, the same transducer is nearly always used for both generation and detection of ultrasound. The transducer axis should be perpendicular to the interface within a few degrees, otherwise the reflected pulse will miss the transducer. In Doppler measurements, separate transducers are used. Special transducer probes have been designed for ophthalmic and intravascular examinations. The latter involves a fiber excited at high frequency (e.g., 20 MHz) inserted through a 1-mm diameter catheter into the blood vessel. The probe tip may be scanned mechanically, or a phased array may be used. The image is then reconstructed and displayed.

8.3 DOPPLER ULTRASOUND

Doppler measurements are used to determine the velocity of objects, based on the shift in frequency. Let the applied ultrasound frequency be f_o and the detected wave frequency be f. The change in frequency when the source and detector approach each other with velocity v is

$$f - f_o = f_o \frac{v}{(v_s - v)}, \qquad (8.10a)$$

and if v_s is much greater than v,

$$f - f_o = f_o \frac{v}{v_s} . \tag{8.10b}$$

The frequency f is greater than f_o.

When the source and detector move away from each other,

$$f - f_o = f_o \frac{-v}{v_s - v} \tag{8.11a}$$

or

$$f - f_o = f_o \frac{-v}{v_s} , \tag{8.11b}$$

when v_s is much greater than v, as is usually true. The frequency is decreased. If the ultrasound is reflected off a moving object and then reaches a stationary detector, the object acts first as a moving detector (velocity v) and then as a moving source as it reflects the wave. The frequency shift is doubled,

$$f - f_o = 2f_o \frac{v}{v_s} \tag{8.12}$$

when moving toward the detector, and

$$f - f_o = 2f_o \frac{-v}{v_s} \tag{8.13}$$

when moving away from the detector. These expressions assume perpendicular incidence. If the ultrasound beam is incident at angle θ, replace v by $v \cos \theta$ in the previous expressions.

A Doppler unit is operated with a continuous wave (cw) output, applied to a transducer. The signal from another, usually adjacent, transducer is amplified by an rf amplifier, and beat against the original oscillator in a demodulator to derive a beat frequency, $f - f_o$. The beat frequency is shown in Fig. 8.4. A Doppler ultrasound unit is often used to measure blood flow by reflection off the red blood cells (RBCs). For example, with $f_o = 10$ MHz and the blood velocity $v = 15$ cm/s toward the the ultrasound source, $f - f_o = 2(10)(15)/154,000 = 1.9$ kHz. The difference (beat) frequency is in the audible range. Doppler is also used to measure the fetal heartbeat from the motion of the heart valves.

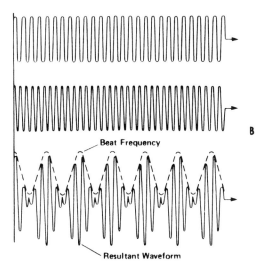

Beat Frequency

B

Resultant Waveform

FIG. 8.4 A beat frequency is observed when transmitted and reflected waves are of nearly the same frequency. (From Bushong, S. C. 1988. *Radiologic science for technologists*. 4th ed. St. Louis: C. V. Mosby.)

8.4 DISPLAY MODES

Diagnostic ultrasound may be displayed in the A-mode (amplitude mode), B-mode (brightness mode), M-mode (motion mode), real-time B-mode, or Doppler mode.

A-Mode

A-mode (see Fig. 8.5) may use one or two transducers. The display is an oscilloscope with the x axis as the time after the source pulse, and the y axis the amplitude of the reflected sound pulse as it reaches the transducer. As with other modes, a sweep gain generator is used so that the detector amplifier gain is increased with time after the source pulse, because the depth of the interface is proportional to the time and the amplitude of the sound pulse is attenuated with depth. A-mode is sometimes used to calibrate other modes. It is also used to test for symmetry in the left and right hemispheres of the brain. In this application, one transducer is placed on the left side of the skull and another on the right side of the skull. A-mode scans are taken for propagation of the ultrasound pulse from left to right, and from right to left. If the hemispheres are symmetrical, the y-axis blip will be in the same position for both directions. Asymmetrical hemispheres may indicate a brain tumor or another disease condition. A-mode, however, is seldom used now.

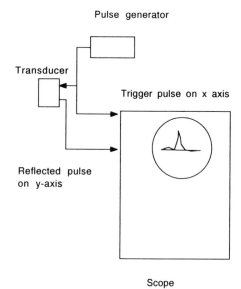

FIG. 8.5 A-mode ultrasound apparatus.

B-Mode

In B-mode (see Fig. 8.6) the x axis is time, but the amplitude of the reflected pulse is indicated by the brightness of a dot. By moving the transducer either linearly or in a motion that describes an arc or a fan, a map can be made the brightness versus time (hence depth) for a large section of the body. A digital scan converter accumulates the information from the many scan lines and prepares it for display on a cathode ray tube. The standard B-mode scan requires the position and angle of the transducer. Linear or rotary transducers (e.g., potentiometers) provide such information. The standard B-mode scan is being replaced by the real-time imaging mode, in which the scanning effect is provided by a phased array transducer. The transducer array is hand held and can be moved to different positions or held at different angles to get a complete picture. Real-time B-mode, probably the most often used mode, is used for abdominal scans and for checking the fetus in pregnant women. A major advantage is that the developing fetus does not receive a dose of ionizing radiation. Figure 8.7 is an example of a diagnostic ultrasound image. It takes training and experience to interpret such images properly.

M-Mode

M-mode (see Fig. 8.8) is used in cardiology, for example. The x axis is a depth axis. The y axis is basically time of day, and the display involves a strip chart recorder, or an equivalent, that displays the dots from the interfaces versus time of day. The M-mode is used for studying the motion of the interface, e.g., in the heart.

Pulse generator

Transducer

Trigger pulse

Brightness

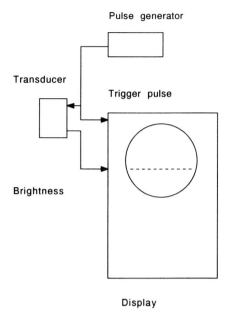

Display

FIG. 8.6 B-mode apparatus for ultrasound imaging.

Doppler Mode

The Doppler mode has already been discussed. The display is usually the audible signal corresponding to the beat frequency, or a sound spectrogram. The Doppler mode is often used to measure the velocity of blood or to indicate a diminution of blood flow because of a partial blockage or stenosis. For example, it can be used to indicate the patency of the carotid artery.

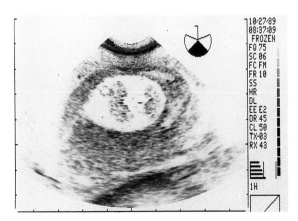

FIG. 8.7 B-mode ultrasound image of twin fetuses. (Courtesy of Siemens Medical Systems, San Ramon, CA.)

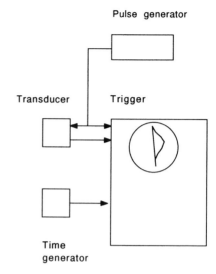

FIG. 8.8   M-mode ultrasonic apparatus.

BIBLIOGRAPHY

Bushong, S. C. 1988. *Radiologic science for technologists*. 4th ed., Chaps. 33–34. St. Louis: C. V. Mosby.

Hendee, W. R. 1979. *Medical radiation physics*, 2d. ed., Chaps. 20–23. Chicago: Year Book Medical Publishers.

West, A. I., ed. 1988. Microsensors and catheter-based imaging technology. Proc. SPIE, Bellingham, WA, Vol. 904, pp. 99–135.

CHAPTER 9

MAGNETIC RESONANCE IMAGING

9.1   PRINCIPLES OF NUCLEAR MAGNETIC RESONANCE

Nuclear magnetic resonance (NMR) is based on deriving a signal from nuclear magnetic moments, initially aligned in a static magnetic field, after excitation with an applied radio frequency (RF) pulse in resonance with the Larmor precession frequency.

An example of a simple NMR system is shown in Fig. 9.1. A sample containing hydrogen is placed between the poles of a magnet that produces a magnetic field, B. The sample is surrounded by a coil of wire that serves as both a transmitting and a receiving antenna. The RF oscillator is tuned in frequency until it is in resonance with the protons. Radio waves of the same frequency are emitted by the sample, inducing small currents in the coil. The amplitude of this signal depends on the number of protons in resonance. Thus the hydrogen density (actually spin density [SD]) can be determined. The SD differs among various tissues.

Larmor Precession Frequency

Certain nuclei have a net magnetic moment, which can be regarded as generated by the spin of the charged nucleus. If proton number Z and neutron number N are odd, the nucleus has integer spin. If $A = Z + N$ is odd, the nucleus has half-integer spin (e.g., ^1H, spin $\frac{1}{2}$). The nucleus acts as a magnetic dipole. If placed in a strong magnetic field, a small fraction (on the order of 10^{-5}) of the nuclei become aligned because of the magnetic force on the dipole. The larger the number of aligned nuclei, the greater the NMR signal. The magnetic moment does not align itself with the magnetic field; instead,

SIMPLE NMR SPECTROMETER

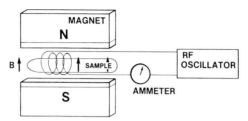

FIG. 9.1 Diagram of a simple NMR spectrometer. (Courtesy of E. McFarland, University of California, Santa Barbara.)

the nucleus wobbles or precesses around the direction of the magnetic field, like a gyroscope or top, as illustrated in Fig. 9.2. The frequency of precession is the Larmor frequency,

$$\omega = 2\pi f = \gamma B_0, \tag{9.1}$$

where B_0 is the strength of the static magnetic field (in tesla, $T = 10{,}000$ gauss), and γ is the gyromagnetic ratio (in megahertz per tesla). The gyromagnetic ratio is a property of each nucleus, and the values for some nuclei are given in Table 9.1. The table also lists the relative abundance of the isotope in the natural element, and the relative magnetic resonance imaging (MRI) sensitivity. Present MRI systems use the proton because of its abundance in tissue and the relatively large MR signal. Research on detection of other nuclei, particularly ^{31}P, is currently under way.

The energy of the magnetic dipole represented by the spinning nucleus depends on its orientation relative to the magnetic field. By quantum mechanics, the spin may be either parallel to the magnetic field vector (pointing toward the north pole), or antiparallel (pointing toward the south pole) in the B_0 field. The energy of the protons with spins pointing north is slightly less than that of protons with spins pointing south, and the energy difference is proportional to the applied field B:

$$\Delta E = (\gamma h/2\pi)B, \tag{9.2}$$

where h is Planck's constant.

If an RF field of frequency $\nu = \Delta E/h$ is applied, usually as a pulse, the parallel protons will absorb energy and point in the antiparallel direction. This energy is soon radiated as RF waves of the same frequency, as the spins return to equilibrium, and it is this resonant radiation that constitutes the signal in NMR.

SPINNING TOP SUBJECTED TO HORIZONTAL FORCE F_x

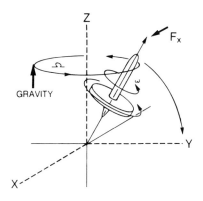

SPINNING PROTON SUBJECTED TO HORIZONTAL FIELD B_x
FROM RF COIL

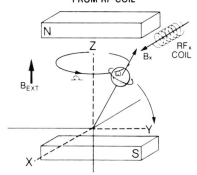

FIG. 9.2   Precession of a spinning gyroscope under gravity and the magnetic moment under an applied field. (Courtesy of E. McFarland, University of California, Santa Barbara.)

TABLE 9.1   NMR Properties of Selected Nuclei

Nuclide	Relative Abundance (%)	Relative Imaging Sensitivity	γ (MHz/T)
^{1}H	99.9	1	43
^{2}H	0.015	91.7×10^{-3}	6.5
^{13}C	1.11	0.016	11
^{19}F	100	0.83	40
^{23}Na	100	0.093	11
^{31}P	100	0.066	17
^{39}K	93.1	5.1×10^{-4}	2

Relaxation Time Constants

In addition to the spin density, samples and tissues vary in their magnetic relaxation times, T_1 and T_2 (time constants). Relaxation is the return to equilibrium following a magnetic perturbation such as from the oscillator RF pulse, as seen in Fig. 9.3. T_1 and T_2 depend on the physical state of the sample (solid or liquid), because of the internal fields. For solids, especially crystalline lattices, the internal fields are relatively strong and fixed in position. For liquids, the internal fields are weak and rapidly fluctuating. T_1 is called the spin-lattice, longitudinal, or thermal relaxation time. It measures the time it takes for the sample to become polarized in the applied magnetic field. A liquid rapidly polarizes because the protons make many collisions with their

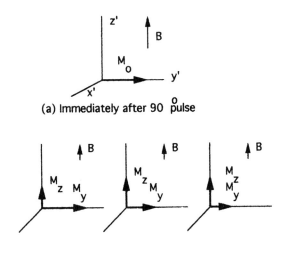

(a) Immediately after 90° pulse

(b) During recovery M_z grows slowly as M_y decays rapidly

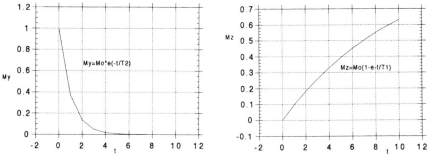

FIG. 9.3 Transverse and longitudinal recovery after 90° pulse. (Courtesy of E. McFarland, University of California, Santa Barbara.)

neighbors per unit time, and T_1 is typically short (milliseconds). A solid polarizes with a long time constant T_1 (seconds).

T_2 is called the spin-spin, transverse, or dephasing relaxation time. It is called the transverse time constant because it applies to the net magnetization perpendicular to B_0, M_{xy}. Part of the NMR technique is that the magnetization is changed from along B_0 to some angle to it, often 90° (hence in the xy-plane with B_0 along the z-axis) or 180°, by application of the RF pulse. Because of local inhomogeneities from neighboring nuclei, the individual magnetic moments become dephased as their precession frequencies are slightly different. This dephasing is a characteristic of T_2 relaxation. If the inhomogeneities are due to an inhomogeneous applied magnetic field, the time constant is called T_2^*. Typically, T_2 is shorter than T_1.

Tissue Properties

Values of SD, T_1, and T_2 for various tissues are listed in Table 9.2 and plotted in Fig. 9.4. The averages for soft tissue are $T_1 = 600$ ms, and $T_2 = 30$ ms. Bone mineral does not emit electromagnetic radiation because it has no hydrogen, but bones contain marrow that does contain hydrogen, and are covered by soft tissue. In NMR, there is no signal from a flowing fluid such as blood or from moving tissue generally, because the magnetic nuclei move out of the field where the signal is generated.

Figure 9.4 also plots the x-ray attenuation coefficient μ in Hounsfield units. NMR provides better differentiation between soft tissues, because of the 20 to 40 percent difference in SD, T_1, and T_2, as compared with the 1 percent difference in μ. Contrast in MRI can be improved even more by using a paramagnetic contrast agent such as a gadolinium-diethylamine triamine pentaacetic acid (DPTA)-meglumine. A contrast agent may modify the field experienced by protons, or may itself be detected. Another advantage of MRI is that it gives a tomographic image like that of computed tomography (CT). A disadvantage is the low signal/noise ratio.

TABLE 9.2 NMR Properties of Various Tissues

Tissue	Relative SD	T_1 (ms)	T_2 (ms)
Water	100	2700	2700
Skeletal muscle	79	720	55
Cardiac muscle	80	725	60
Liver	71	290	50
Fat	360	30	
Bone	<12	<100	<10
Spleen	79	570	
Kidney	81	505	50
Brain (gray matter)	84	405	105
Brain (white matter)	70	345	65

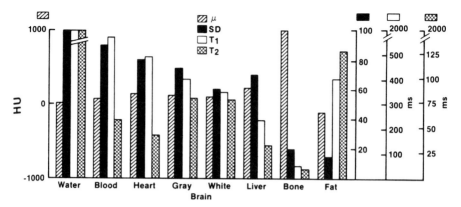

FIG. 9.4 Comparison of x-ray attenuation coefficient (in Hounsfield units) with MRI properties SD, T_1, and T_2. (From Bushong, S. C. 1988. *Radiologic science for technologists*. 4th ed. St. Louis: C. V. Mosby.)

Free Induction Decay

The number of nuclei of a given type is found by measuring the number with an appropriate Larmor frequency. If an RF pulse of the proper frequency is applied, the energy is transferred to the nuclei with that Larmor frequency, a process called *resonance*. The nuclear spin axes are caused to rotate through some angle, usually 90° or 180°, by the RF coil, as shown in Fig. 9.2, and the nuclei are caused to precess in phase. When the RF excitation pulse is removed, the nuclei relax to equilibrium more or less exponentially and emit an RF wave, a process called free induction decay (FID). The intensity versus time information is converted into intensity versus frequency by means of a Fourier transform operation, as shown in Fig. 9.5. The signal is proportional to the SD, and hence to the concentration of protons (or other nuclei). The rate of decay of the FID signal amplitude is a combination of T_1 and T_2.

9.2 MAGNETIC RESONANCE IMAGING

Gradient Fields

MRI differs from classical NMR in that an image is obtained. The image is derived by adding a small, spatially varying, linear gradient magnetic field (B_1) to the main static field (B_0) along the z-axis (the cranio-caudad axis of the patient), the x-axis, and the y-axis. Each voxel (volume element), $\Delta x \Delta y \Delta z$, has a slightly different Larmor frequency for the proton, providing information on the net B field and, hence, position. By rotating the gradient field, multiple spectra can be obtained as a function of angle, and a tomographic image can be reconstructed as in CT, or in any place including a sagittal plane. Instead of an x-ray attenuation coefficient, one obtains SD, T_1, or T_2. Filtered

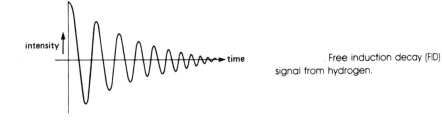

intensity ↑

→ time

Free induction decay (FID)
signal from hydrogen.

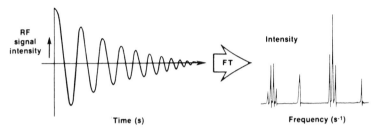

RF
signal ↑
intensity

FT

Intensity

Time (s)

Frequency (s⁻¹)

FIG. 9.5 Fourier transform of a free induction decay signal in an NMR spectrum. (From Bushong, S. C. 1988. *Radiologic science for technologists.* 4th ed. St. Louis: C. V. Mosby.)

back projection and similar techniques may be applied, but the preferred technique for MRI is spin echo. Resolution is 0.5 to 1.0 mm.

Spin Echo

The spin echo is a burst of RF waves emitted after a delay, when the protons are excited by a combination of a 90° pulse and one or more 180° pulses, as shown in Fig. 9.6, which is plotted in the rotational frame (precessing at the Larmor frequency). The 90° pulse is RF excitation along the x-axis for long enough to shift the magnetization vector, M, into the y-direction from the z-direction. The 180° pulse is twice as long and is applied after a delay time τ_2. After the 90° pulse, dephasing occurs because of the varying local magnetic fields encountered, resulting in different rates of precession of the transverse magnetic vectors making up M. When the 180° pulse is applied, the vectors are reversed and eventually reestablish coherence (vectors in-phase). An RF pulse is emitted—the spin echo, as seen in Fig. 9.7. The amplitude of the echo indicates the number of protons involved and how well they remain in-phase (T_2) despite inhomogeneities in the applied external magnetic field. The frequency of the spin echo indicates the strength of the local magnetic field, and hence position, as explained in the preceding section on gradient fields. By changing the magnetic field gradients during the two pulses, different planes can be read out. The time between pulses can be varied for T_2 weighting or T_1 weighting.

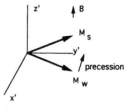

(a) Dephasing transverse magnetization
(Ms in stroger field and precessing at
higher rate than Mw)

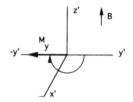

(b) Rotation of My component following
180 degree RF pulse

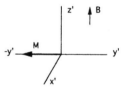

FIG. 9.6 Dephasing and rephasing after 90 and 180 degree pulses. (Courtesy of E. McFarland, University of California, Santa Barbara.)

(c) Coherence reestablished

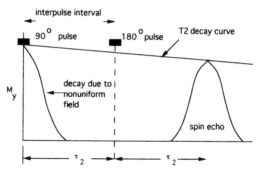

FIG. 9.7 The spin echo following 90 and 180 degree pulses. (Courtesy of E. McFarland, University of California, Santa Barbara.)

9.3 MRI SYSTEMS AND IMAGES

An MRI system consists of a magnet assembly, an RF transmitter and receiver, a computer, and a display device. The magnet assembly includes a high-strength magnet for the B_0 field, shim coils to improve the homogeneity of the B_0 field, and gradient coils. The magnets are shown in Fig. 9.8.

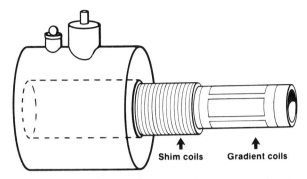

FIG. 9.8 Magnet coils and dewar of a magnetic resonance imaging unit. (From Bushong, S. C. 1988. *Radiologic science for technologists*, 4th ed. St. Louis: C. V. Mosby.)

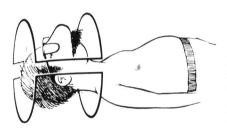

FIG. 9.9 Saddle-shaped RF probe for excitation and reception of the MRI signal. (From Bushong, S. C. 1988. *Radiologic science for technologists*. St. Louis: C. V. Mosby.)

The main magnet is nearly always a superconductor, now of the type that must be cooled to liquid helium temperature (4 K). It is contained in a dewar and surrounded by liquid nitrogen (77 K) and superinsulation. Sources of liquid helium and liquid nitrogen are provided, either externally or by a cryogenic refrigerator. A superconducting magnet coil can generate a magnetic field of some 1 to 2 T over a region large enough to image a section of the body. The requirement for homogeneity is very strict: about 50 parts per million. Homogeneity is improved by a series of resistive shim coils, each with its own power supply. The currents are adjusted while mapping the magnetic field.

Figure 9.8 includes a schematic diagram of the X and Y gradient coils. The Z gradient coils are coils near each end of the main magnet, lying in the *x-y* plane (perpendicular to the *z*-axis, the patient's cranio-caudad axis). Energizing the Z coils selects a transverse layer for imaging. The shim coils and gradient coils actually lie inside the bore of the main magnet.

The RF probe or antenna is located inside the gradient coils. A typical saddle-shaped probe is shown in Fig. 9.9. The same probe is used to excite the nuclei and receive the signal radiated as the nuclei return to equilibrium. The frequency is the Larmor frequency, 86 MHz for protons in a field of 2 T. This lies within the TV band.

The MRI unit is not likely to interfere with TV, but TV can interfere with

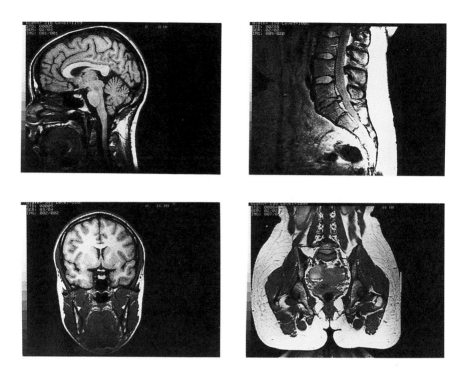

FIG. 9.10 Magnetic resonance images. (Courtesy of General Electric MR Development Center, Milwaukee.) (*Upper left*) Image of head demonstrating excellent soft-tissue contrast and fine anatomic detail, 3 mm thick slice, 1.5 Tesla. (*Upper right*) Image of lumbar spine in sagittal plane showing herniated disc at L5-S1 level. (*Lower left*) Image of head in coronal plane showing pituitary fossa. (*Lower right*) Image of abdomen showing psoas muscle, uterus, bladder, pelvic bone marrow. Bright area is a pelvic cyst.

the detection of the weak MRI signal. Therefore, the MRI unit is housed in a Faraday cage (wire-mesh electromagnetic shield). Electrical penetrations into the room are fitted with electrical filters, and DC lighting should be used. Magnetic devices should be avoided. Ferromagnetic material in the vicinity can perturb the magnetic field of the MRI unit, not only outside but also inside the magnet assembly. Thus construction must avoid the use of iron or steel. For example, steel reinforcing rods in the walls may be replaced by rods of polyvinyl chloride. Distance, hence lower field strength, is needed to protect certain devices from the fringe magnetic field of the MRI units. For example, neither the patient nor the operator should carry credit cards or wear an analog watch. The next most sensitive devices are computers and disk drives, followed by video cameras and cathode ray tubes, heart pacemakers and image intensifiers, and a CT scanner or nuclear medicine camera. There is no known biological effect of the magnetic field (or RF) in MRI systems, and, of course, there is no ionizing radiation.

Figure 9.10 is a group of tomographic images taken with an MRI machine. The appearance of the image can be changed by the selection of the RF pulse sequence, as can the proportions of SD, T_1, and T_2.

The large variation of SD, T_1, and T_2 provides very good contrast between tissues, enough to distinguish various soft tissues. Individual parameters can be used, or the T_1-weighted SD image, T_2-weighted SD image, and so forth, can be constructed. It is even possible to achieve image contrast reversal, or a null region where all contrast is lost. Contrast between tissues of differing T_1 can be enhanced by adjusting the pulse repetition rate. Spin echo is a method of imaging with T_2. Different pulse repetition rates and 90° versus 180° pulses should be applied to obtain the best image for the tissues involved. More information may be found in Valk, and colleagues, pages 53–83, and in Young, pages 51–54 and 151 (listed in the Bibliography of this chapter).

BIBLIOGRAPHY

Bushong, S. C. 1988. *Radiologic science for technologists.* 4th ed. Chaps. 33–34. St. Louis: C. V. Mosby, pp. 595–634.

Valk, J., C. MacLean, and P. R. Algra. 1985. *Basic principles of nuclear magnetic imaging.* New York: Elsevier.

Patz, S. 1986. Basic physics of nuclear magnetic resonance. *Cardiovascular and Interventional Radiology* 8:225–237.

Young, S. W. 1984. *Nuclear magnetic resonance imaging.* New York: Raven Press.

APPENDIX A

SAFETY

A.1 ELECTRICAL SAFETY

Continuous availability of electrical power is important for certain lights, life-support instrumentation, and critical monitoring systems. A hospital generally has an emergency generator, often powered by a diesel engine, to supply power within 10 seconds after a power outage.

Electrical safety is an important concern regarding current passing through the heart, which may cause fibrillation and thus loss of pumping. The current may also affect the central nervous system (CNS), interfering with nerve conduction and causing consequent dysfunction. Such a hazard may be considered either as a macroshock or a microshock. A *macroshock* is one in which the current flows through the skin and tissue before and after encountering the heart. It involves currents generally greater then 1 mA applied to the intact dry skin, which has an epidermal resistivity of 100,000 to 300,000 Ω/cm^2. Wet skin may have a resistivity of 1 percent of the dry skin value. Thus the minimum resistance across intact skin is a nominal 1000 Ω. The internal resistance of the tissues is generally taken as 500 Ω. In current flow along the body's vertical axis, 10 percent may flow through the heart. As to current flow along a horizontal axis, 3 percent may flow through the heart. Microampere currents applied directly across the heart constitute a *microshock*. The currents may be applied by wires or by conducting fluid in a catheter.

The threshold of fibrillation, as for a microshock, depends on the physiological condition of the heart and is also affected by the electrode position, size, and current density; time in the electrocardiogram (ECG) cycle (T wave is most sensitive); and duration of application. Standards codes generally limit the current to about 10 to 20 μA to avoid fibrillation.

Macroshock effects include perception current, let-go current, and fibrillatory current. The perception current is the minimum current that can be perceived by the subject. It differs between men and women and depends on frequency. It is generally between 1 and 2 mA. The let-go current is the current above which the subject cannot let go of the conductor, because of tetanic contraction of the forearm muscles. It is generally about 10 mA for women and 16 mA for men. The current in which heart fibrillation occurs in 95 percent of the subjects for a 1-second duration is between 185 mA for adults and 60 mA for children. Safe, nonfibrillatory currents are 116 mA for adults and 52 mA for children. Currents greater than 2A to 6A may cause cardiac arrest, paralysis, and deep burns.

Codes are revised from time to time; therefore, the latest codes for electrical wiring should be consulted or a knowledgeable contractor chosen. Few installations use flammable anesthetics anymore, but if a flammable anesthetic is present, the electrical equipment must be designed to prevent sparks. The usual requirements for patient protection against shock call for grounding all electrical equipment and other conducting objects, such as tray tables, which could come in contact with the patient. The equipment is powered by a three-wire cord and plug (hot, neutral, and ground). Color coding of plugs is as follows: gold for hot, white for neutral, and green for ground. The ground wire, of at least a no. 10 AWG size, is connected to the earth ground of the building through the structural steel or cold-water piping. All equipment and other conductors near a patient should be grounded at one point, to avoid differences in potential because of leakage currents. The grounding system protects the patient against macroshock in event of an electrical fault, and against microshock resulting from leakage current through insulators or electronic components. The leakage current should be measured by the voltage across a 1000 Ω resistor or with a voltmeter of 1000 Ω input resistance, and in new construction the potential should not exceed 20 mV.

Another solution is to use isolated power supplies, the equipment being powered from the secondary of a transformer. A line-isolation monitor may be installed to monitor the leakage current or fault current to ground, and to sound an alarm if it becomes excessive. Another device is a ground-fault interrupter, which monitors the difference in current between the hot and neutral wires and trips a circuit breaker if the current gets too high.

A.2 OPTICAL SAFETY

Sources of electromagnetic radiation, including ultraviolet (UV), visible light (VIS), and infrared (IR), may present a hazard to the cornea or retina of the eye and to the skin. The site and amount of damage depends on the power, spot area (hence, power density), depth of penetration and absorption fraction (hence, wavelength), duration of exposure, and pulse width (if not continuous wave). Because of the high power density capability of lasers, they are of particular concern.

Most of the action of optical radiation is thermal, resulting in denaturation or coagulation of protein and inactivation of enzymes. An exception is the photochemical reaction of the actinic UV from 200 to 320 nm. The response is a "sunburn" or photokeratinitis, also known as snowblindness or welder's flash, occurring with a threshold of about 4 mJ/cm². A similar effect (erythema) occurs on the skin, with a threshold of 1 W/cm² for exposures greater than 10 seconds for the CO_2 laser). Thermal effects depend on the pulse width relative to the thermal diffusion time (on the order of 1 ms) and on the energy deposited, and hence on the duration of exposure.

Far UV and far IR are absorbed in the cornea. Near UV is absorbed in the cornea and lens. The cornea and lens transmit most of the visible and near IR (400 to 1400 nm), and the radiation can be focused to a small spot on the retina, where about half is absorbed in the pigmented retinal epithelium.

Although the eye is the principal organ of concern, the skin should also be considered. The worst condition for the eye is produced by staring into the beam, but head adversion and blinking tend to reduce the danger in practice. Diffusely reflected light is a danger with high-power lasers, and specular or mirror reflection is nearly as dangerous as looking into the beam.

The potential for injury in the VIS and near IR is increased because the light can be focused by the lens to a very small diameter. The image diameter at the retina, for small angles, is

$$d_r = D_L f_e / r, \qquad (A.1)$$

where d_r is the focused spot diameter, D_L is the diameter of the light source, f_e is the effective focal length (1.7 cm for the normal, emmetropic eye), and r is the distance from source to eye. However, the spot diameter cannot be less than that allowed by diffraction:

$$d_r(\text{min}) = 2.44 \ \lambda \ f_e / d_e, \qquad (A.2)$$

where λ is the wavelength and d_e is the pupil diameter. For $\lambda = 500$ nm, $d_e = 3$ mm, $d_r(\text{min})$ is 6.9 μm. The relationship between the source radiance L and the retinal irradiance E_r is

$$E_r = 0.27 \ d_p^2 \ \tau \ L, \qquad (A.3)$$

where τ is the transmittance of the ocular media, and the pupil diameter d_p is given in centimeters. The pupil diameter will vary from about 0.1 cm in bright light to about 0.7 cm in dim light. The transmittance is nearly 1.0 in the 450 to 900 nm band, but decreases outside that band.

Laser safety standards are based on biological response versus dose and dose rate, so that no effect is anticipated in any subject. The dose limits and safety standards are set by the Bureau of Radiological Health (BRH) of the federal Food and Drug Administration, the American Conference of Governmental Industrial Hygienists (ACGIH), and the American National Standards Institute (ANSI). The allowable energy entering the eye is set in ANSI Z-136, depending on pulse duration. In the VIS, below 2×10^{-5} seconds, this is 2×10^{-7} J. Above 10 seconds it is 5.5×10^{-3} J, and the limit increases linearly (on a log-log plot) between these times. A higher dose is allowed at longer wavelengths. Formulas for exposure limits are given versus wavelength, for certain durations, in Sliney and Worbarsht (Tables 8-1, 8-2, and 8-3, pages 262–263), listed in the Bibliography at the end of this Appendix. These are derived from standard ANSI Z-136.1-1986, for direct viewing of a laser beam, for diffuse reflection into the eye, and for irradiation of the skin.

The hazard produced by lasers is determined by the manufacturer, and each laser is classified according to its risk or, approximately, by its power as defined by the BRH. Each class has certain controls or safety features:

Class I: Minimal risk, very low power (such as μW GaAs laser diodes). No special controls

Class II: Low risk, low power. Risk is from staring into the beam, or pointing the beam so that it hits another person's eye. Requires protective housing with safety interlock, keyswitch to prevent unauthorized operation, emission indicator (visual or audible) when laser is on, shutter or attenuator on the beam aperture, and a caution label

Class III: Moderate risk, medium power. Injury occurs within the blink delay time (0.25 seconds). Not hazardous for diffuse reflection or to skin, controls same as Class II, plus danger (or caution) label, and remote control connector

Class IV: High risk, high power. Injury to eye even within blink, direct or diffuse reflection. Injury to skin. Controls same as Class III, plus localized enclosure or light-tight room with opaque doors, warning-light outside door, and danger labels and signs

Persons working within the controlled area should wear protective goggles. These come in different colors, with low transmission at the laser wavelength and higher transmission at other wavelengths so that the wearer is not effectively blind. If the beam could injure skin or start a fire, the location of the beam should be apparent (e.g., by mixing a HeNe laser beam with an invisible CO_2 laser beam), fire-resistant backstop should be provided, as well as suitable shielding between the laser and personnel.

Many medical lasers are Class III, and a few may be Class IV. The precautions taken, besides those discussed, may include the following:

Draping a surgical incision with wet towels
Providing a focusing guide

Minimizing specular reflections

Avoiding use of a combustible anesthetic

Providing an emergency foot switch or hand trigger to shut off the beam

A.3 RADIOLOGICAL SAFETY

Radiological safety is concerned with the hazards of exposure to ionizing radiation, especially x-rays, gamma rays, electrons, and neutrons. A distinction is made between external and internal sources of ionizing radiation. The latter involves radionuclides administered in connection with nuclear medicine procedures or accidentally ingested. External sources include x-ray diagnostic equipment, x-rays or energetic electrons from linacs for radiotherapy, and radioisotopes encapsulated for brachytherapy.

Dose equivalent is given by

$$H = DQ, \tag{A.1}$$

where D is the absorbed dose discussed earlier in Chapters 6 and 7 on radiology and nuclear medicine, and Q is the quality factor that takes into account linear energy transfer (LET), the density of ionizations along the path of the particle (including secondary electrons from x-rays and gamma rays). For x-rays, gamma rays, and electrons, LET is small and $Q = 1$. For fast neutrons, recoil protons are generated by neutron collisions, their LET is large, and $Q = 10$ or so, depending on the energy. Slow neutrons interact, mainly by absorption in hydrogen, to produce gamma rays. They also react by the $^{14}N(n, p)^{14}C$ reaction. The Q for slow neutrons is about 5.

Dose equivalents from different types of radiation add to give a measure of the total hazard. The absorbed dose or dose equivalent of x-rays and gamma rays can be measured with a tissue-equivalent ionization chamber, such as shown in Fig. 6.27. For radiation protection purposes, the dose rate is measured with a portable battery-powered instrument, a survey meter. The dose equivalent for neutrons is usually measured with a ^3He proportional counter, with the neutrons being moderated or slowed down by a cylinder of polyethylene surrounding the counter tube. The diameter of the polyethylene is chosen so that the overall response is similar to that of the human body, in terms of dose equivalent versus neutron energy. The neutron survey meter can also be made portable and battery operated. The units of dose equivalent are sievert (1 Sv = 1 Gy for x-rays) or rem (1 rem = 1 rad = 0.01 Gy for x-rays).

The dose received from internally administered radionuclides is not easily determined. Often bioassays are used, for example, for detection of any radioactivity in urine. Another approach is to count gamma rays emanating from the body in a shielded room with a large gamma-ray detector (whole-body counter).

The biological effects of whole-body irradiation at high levels include damage to sensitive tissues such as bone marrow, the lining of the gastrointestinal tract, and even the central nervous system (CNS). Symptoms include a decline in number of blood cells, nausea and vomiting, and even neurological dysfunctions such as convulsions if the dose is high enough (the acute radiation syndrome). The subject may become very sick and even die, especially if not provided with adequate medical treatment. However, the threshold for observable blood cell changes is about 50 rem. The mean threshold for death is some 450 rem. Radiation sickness increases in severity and requires longer recovery with doses between about 100 and 450 rem. Note that this applies to whole-body irradiation, especially to the bone marrow, the gastrointestinal tract, and the brain. Doses on the order of 200 rem per treatment, and a few thousand rem total, are given locally to tumors in radiotherapy. No deaths have been reported, and radiation sickness is minimal in such cases.

When a dose may be delivered over many days at low levels, the principal effects of concern are mutations to the germ cells (sperm and ova) and carcinogenesis. It is assumed that there is no threshold for these effects, and the rate of mutation or probability of carcinogenesis is proportional to the total dose accumulated, independent of the rate at which it is delivered. The Committee on the Biological Effects of Ionizing Radiation (BEIR) has found that the spontaneous mutation rate is doubled with a dose between 20 and 200 rem. The risks of carcinogenesis are summarized in Table A.1. Risk depends on age, the young being more susceptible than adults. The latent period refers to the time between radiation exposure and diagnosis of the cancer. It may reflect the effect of cumulative exposure and repair, or the time for a single cell to grow into a tumor large enough to be detected. Typically, there follows a plateau interval, in which the cancers are expressed, and then a decrease to normal levels.

These dose rates can be put somewhat in perspective by considering the natural dose rate of about 100 mrem/y from cosmic rays and radioactive minerals in soil or in buildings. The natural background radiation dose rate increases with altitude (because of less air shielding objects from cosmic rays)

TABLE A.1   Radiation Carcinogenesis

Age	Type	Latent Period (years)	Plateau (years)	Risk deaths year − 10⁶ persons − rem
In utero	Leukemia	0	10	25
	All other	0	10	25
0–9 y	Leukemia	2	25	2.0
	All other	15	Life	1.0
10+ y	Leukemia	2	25	1.0
	All other	15	Life	5.0

and varies with the composition of the materials. People are also exposed to radiation from the ^{40}K isotope of potassium in their own bodies, and from any radionuclides in their food and drink. Medical procedures add another 100 mrem/y to the dose received by the average American. Of course, specific medical procedures such as a computed tomography (CT) scan or a nuclear medicine scan will give much more radiation to an individual. Doses to patients from medical procedures are not controlled by the government but left up to the physician, who considers the importance of diagnosis or treatment versus risk posed by the dose. In any case, the dose should be minimized. Doses to medical personnel, such as x-ray technicians or nuclear medicine technologists, are controlled.

The basic limit for occupational exposure is 5 rem/y or 2.5 mrem/h. There is a desire to reduce this level by another factor of 10, to some 0.2 mrem/h for the general public and for occupational exposure, following the philosophy of ALARA (as low as reasonably achievable). In any case, the x-ray technician retreats to a shielded area while exposing the patient to radiation. Nuclear medicine personnel should take precautions to avoid ingesting any radiopharmaceutical material.

If the external dose rate is high, the dose can be decreased by distance (the flux density drops off as $1/r^2$ for a point isotropic source) by limiting the time near the source and by interposing shielding (e.g., lead or concrete for x-rays or gamma rays). The dose from internally administered radionuclides is limited by injecting only as much activity as will be needed for the procedure, by getting all the information from one injection, by choosing radionuclides with little beta (electron) emission energy, and, if possible, by choosing a radiopharmaceutical with short radiological and biological half-life. Accidental ingestion of a radiopharmaceutical is prevented by wearing rubber gloves, not drinking or eating in the area, not smoking or applying cosmetics, keeping the air clean, and disposing of radioactive material properly. Frequent surveys should be made of countertops and other surfaces to detect radioactive contamination. Such surfaces should be covered with absorbent paper with a plastic film backing. "Radioactive Material Caution" signs should be posted in the area.

BIBLIOGRAPHY

National Research Council. 1972. *BEIR Report: The effects on populations of exposure to low levels of ionizing radiation*, Washington: National Academy of Sciences.

Profio, A. E. 1979. *Radiation shielding and dosimetry*. New York: John Wiley & Sons.

Sliney, D., and M. Worbarsht. 1980. *Safety with lasers and other optical sources*. New York: Plenum Press.

Wald, A. 1987. Electrical safety in medicine. In *Handbook of bioengineering*, ed. R. Skalak and S. Chien. New York: McGraw-Hill, pp. 34.1–34.20.

APPENDIX B

TISSUE AND ANIMAL EXPERIMENTATION

This section addresses experimentation with cells, tissues (live or dead), organ preparations, and the intact, living animal.

Experiments with cells are performed in many biomedical investigations. An example is the determination of the cell survival curve, the fraction of clonogenic (reproducing) cells left after irradiation with a certain dose of radiation.

Not all cells divide and reproduce well in culture or in the mature animal, but malignant cancer cells do. Generally, they are grown on a culture medium in a Petri dish, or in a flat bottle mounted slantwise. The culture medium is usually based on agar, for solidity, and incorporates the essential nutrients as well as a buffer to control pH. Such culture media are available commercially from laboratory supply houses. A small amount of penicillin may be added to suppress bacterial infection. The Petri dishes or bottles are held at a constant temperature (37°C for human cells) in an incubator, perhaps in a CO_2-enriched atmosphere.

In radiation biology, 20 to 50 single cells are inoculated at several places on the medium and the cultures allowed to grow until the cell colonies can be counted with the naked eye. At least 50 divisions are considered necessary for clonogenic survival. The control (nonirradiated) dish is evaluated to determine the *plating efficiency*—the fraction of cells inoculated that grow into colonies—which may be 50 to 90 percent. The remaining dishes are exposed to a graded series of doses, and the fraction of cells surviving (growing clonogenic colonies) is evaluated, corrected for the plating efficiency, and plotted as the logarithm of the cell-survival fraction against dose, as shown in Fig. B.1.

The curve often shows a shoulder followed by an exponential decline. The

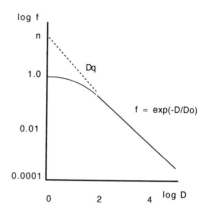

FIG. B.1 Surviving fraction f vs. dose in grays.

shoulder has been attributed to repair of sublethal damage and to the multitarget single-hit model where several sites or targets must be altered by the radiation. If the straight-line portion of the logarithmic curve is extrapolated back to zero dose, one gets n, the extrapolation number, which may be interpreted as the target multiplicity. The intersection of the extrapolated curve with a surviving fraction of 1.0 gives the quasithreshold dose, D_q. The slope of the straight-line portion is given by $1/D_o$, where D_o is the dose required to reduce the surviving fraction by $1/e = 37$ percent. The quantities are related by $D_q = D_o \ln n$.

Tissue specimens are often used in experiments. These are dead, and the properties of dead tissues may be different from those in the in vivo state because of aging or loss of moisture, for example. Such specimens will not be provided with the same amount of blood, especially flowing, oxygenated blood. Major changes are minimized by quick-freezing the specimens and making the measurements as soon as they thaw to near room temperature. Slow freezing is to be avoided because of the growth of ice crystals that can disrupt the cells.

Live tissue specimen and organ preparations are seldom used because of the difficulty of supplying oxygenated blood and nutrients to them. However, a similar preparation can be achieved by isolating a part of a living animal, e.g., the ear of a rabbit or the cheek pouch of a hamster. The area of interest can be sealed off in a chamber with windows and methods of applying the experimental device, while allowing the blood to circulate.

Many experiments are done in animals before an experimental device is applied to human beings. This may or may not involve surgery. There are many regulations that must be followed, and the proposed experiments are subject to review and approval by the institution's animal research committee. The major points to consider are as follows:

1. The procedure should be necessary, and good scientific data must be obtained.

2. Pain and suffering to the animal must be minimized, e.g., by the use of anesthetics. If the animal will survive a surgical procedure, sterile techniques and good surgical practice should be observed.

3. If pain cannot be prevented, the ethics of the experiment should be scrutinized.

4. Only as many animals should be used as are really necessary to obtain good data, including statistical precision. Rodents, especially mice and rats, bred for the purpose of scientific research, should be used if possible. Rare and expensive higher animals such as primates (monkeys) should not be used unless absolutely necesary. The use of dogs and cats obtained from pounds raises the question of using pets, and is also best avoided if possible. Some experiments are done on cattle and sheep (e.g., in development of the artificial heart), pigs (which have anatomical features similar to humans), and rabbits (especially for experiments involving the eyes).

BIBLIOGRAPHY

Alpen, E. L. 1990. *Radiation biophysics*. Englewood Cliffs, N.J.: Prentice-Hall.

Kruse, P. F., and M. K. Patterson. 1973. *Tissue culture*. New York: Academic Press.

APPENDIX C

HUMAN EXPERIMENTATION

Experiments with human subjects raise a number of ethical questions. Yet it is undoubtedly true that the first applications of a new medical device, let alone new drugs, must be considered experimental. The approval of new medical devices rests with the Food and Drug Administration (FDA) in the United States. Experimental trials must also be approved by the human subjects committee of the institution so involved.

The first trials of a new medical device may be approved under an IND (investigatory new device) exemption. Generally, this requires an application to the FDA, accompanied by records of experiments on animals or previous experience with similar devices. The aim of the FDA is to protect the public by requiring proof of safety and efficacy (that is, that the device does what is claimed for it). Another approach for occasional application is "compassionate use," for cases in which other established procedures have failed and the new technique offers some promise.

Eventually the FDA will require a formal application for a protocol, in which a specific model of the device is applied to a specific medical problem. A different protocol is required for each medical problem. FDA approval of protocols requires a great many records documenting the experimental application of a device, perhaps by a number of investigators. The safety and efficacy of the protocol procedure must be addressed, and follow-up examinations may be required to determine whether there are any long-term or delayed side effects or failure of the procedure in the long term. Because it would be unethical to deprive a patient of a standard treatment that might help him or her, controlled blind studies are difficult to arrange. Such studies are important, however, to avoid investing in a procedure whose good effect is actually due to something else (e.g., the placebo effect) while the procedure itself is ineffective. Frequently, an experimental procedure is combined with an established procedure and any improvement noted. In some cases patients who have similar medical conditions may be compared, with some randomly assigned to the established procedure and others randomly assigned to the experimental procedure, if the difference between the outcome of the procedures is not great. This process is lengthy and may be quite expensive.

The crux of human experimentation and application of experimental devices and procedures is competent and informed consent. The experimental procedure or device is described in writing in layman's language in the Consent Form. The anticipated medical benefits, and any possible side effects together with the risk, are also included in the Consent Form. The patient has to be reassured that he or she will receive the best possible medical attention, regardless of whether he or she consents to the experimental investigation. Thus the patient must be informed of the proposed procedure and must sign the form to indicate consent. Those whose mental competency to understand the procedure, such as retarded persons, should be omitted from such procedures unless a legal guardian or parent consents for him or her. Persons, such as prisoners, whose free will to chose or not to chose inclusion in the study is questionable, are also best omitted unless they really want to cooperate. In evaluating the benefit versus risk, it is desirable that the application of the new device helps the person who is exposed to it. In some cases, a patient will volunteer to be included in order to help humanity, even if direct benefit to the him or her is problematic.

An example of an Informed Consent form is given in Exhibit C.1.

EXHIBIT C.1   Informed Consent

Consent to Participate in a Clinical Research Study

Study Title: A Randomized, Phase III Study of the Safety and Efficacy of Photodynamic Therapy (PDT) Utilizing PHOTOFRIN II (Dihematoporphyrin Ethers [DHE]) versus Observation Treatment in the Prophylaxis of Transitional Cell Carcinoma of the Urinary Bladder

Protocol: D73 P32 T

Informed Consent

1. I understand that I have cancer of the urinary bladder. Treatment for this disease may include removal of the tumor tissue from the bladder through a cystoscope (transurethral resection [TUR]) and subsequent removal of recurrent tumor tissue as it arises. Following each resection, patients may be closely followed by observation, or an experimental chemotherapeutic agent may be instilled into the bladder. Even when treated in this fashion, some patients have recurrence of the cancer or a progression or spread of the tumor.

This present research study is intended to determine any difference in time to reappearance, if any, of bladder tumors following TUR in patients with (a) no further treatment other than repeated observation and (b) those who are treated with an experimental procedure called "photodynamic therapy" (PDT) followed by repeated observation. I understand that my assignment to either of these two treatment groups will be determined by chance (randomization) almost equivalent to the toss of a coin.

I understand that if my bladder disease recurs during the observation time of this study, I will be removed immediately from the study and may then be eligible for entry to protocol D73-P31. Once trial exit data are acquired, I will no longer be subjected to tests and procedures as required by this study.

I understand that as long as my bladder disease does not return, I will be required to undergo various tests (described below in this section) to determine my progress at quarterly intervals (every three months) for two years following either injection of PHOTOFRIN II or the initiation of observation (no treatment).

I understand that treatment with photodynamic therapy (PDT) is an experimental therapy for the kind of bladder tumor(s) I have. The therapy consists of the injection of the drug PHOTOFRIN II into one of my veins. Two days after this injection, I will undergo cystoscopy; a fiber attached to a light source will be inserted into my bladder via the cystoscope and the light will be shone for an amount of time suitable for my condition. I will undergo an additional cystoscopy without exposure to light 12 weeks after photodynamic therapy and at quarterly intervals (every 3 months) thereafter for 1 year or until recurrence of my disease, whichever occurs first. The portion of this treatment that is considered experimental is the use of the investigational drug PHOTOFRIN II, followed by the shining of the light into the bladder. I understand that intravenous injections of PHOTOFRIN II or its predecessor, hematoporphyrin derivative (HPD), followed by photoradiation therapy, has already been performed in more than 1500 patients and is currently undergoing tests at a number of medical institutions in the United States and abroad.

I understand that photodynamic therapy may not result in the cure of my cancer.

I understand that to be admitted to this trial I must have undergone a transurethral resection of my bladder tumor(s). Other procedures I will undergo upon entering this study, whether I am treated with PDT or not, are: medical history, physical examination, electrocardiogram (ECG), chest x-ray, measurement of bladder capacity, assessment of urinary symptoms, cystoscopy, biopsies of several bladder sites, and laboratory tests of blood and urine. These procedures will be repeated 12 weeks after randomization to PDT treatment, and, with the exception of blood and urine tests, at all subsequent quarterly evaluations. I will be contacted weekly by telephone regarding urinary symptoms and any adverse experiences. Blood and urine samples will also be taken on the day of light application and 7 days thereafter if I receive PDT therapy.

2. I understand that if I am treated with PHOTOFRIN II, the most likely foreseeable risk or discomfort owing to my participation in this study is an immediate, greatly increased sensitivity of my skin to bright light, either natural (e.g., direct or indirect sunlight) or strong, direct indoor lighting (e.g., direct spotlight, dentist's light), and to radiant heat (e.g., helmet-type hair dryer) for a period of at least 4 to 6 weeks following injection of PHOTOFRIN II. I understand that the doctors and staff conducting this study are aware of this risk I am taking and will take precautions to protect me from sunburn. I understand that I must avoid exposure to bright light. If exposure to sunlight or bright light is unavoidable

during this period, I must cover my skin with clothing (long sleeves, gloves, etc.) and use sunglasses. If these precautions are not undertaken, I understand that a severe sunburn can result in a matter of minutes. Sunscreen lotions have not been proven significantly effective in protecting against sunlight in the photosensitivity produced by PHOTOFRIN II. The method of my periodically testing for continuing hypersensitivity to light will be explained by me by study personnel.

The effects of skin photosensitization and precautions taken to avoid light exposure will be specifically monitored during weeks 2 to 12 in both treated and untreated groups in the study. I will be asked to complete a list of questions prior to injection and at intervals thereafter. The questions will be designed to estimate time spent outdoors in various activities both before and after PDT and document the precautions taken to avoid skin photosensitivity. In addition, I will be asked to administer a self-test for skin photosensitivity via a patch-testing procedure once prior to injection, and at weekly intervals from 2 to 12 weeks after injection of PHOTOFRIN II. I will be asked to keep a diary of weekly events relating to skin photosensitivity, and will also be contacted by the study center weekly and asked to respond to a set of questions designed to elicit information on any occurrences of photosensitivity.

Although no lasting bladder effects have been observed in patients receiving photoradiation therapy to the bladder, there have been cases of patients who have experienced some pain, hematuria (blood in the urine), urinary frequency, and urgency or difficulty in urination, as well as discharge of necrotic debris (dead tissue) within a few days of treatment. These symptoms subsided over a few days. There is a chance that there will be an increased risk of infection as a result of the therapy. Bladder contracture or scarring could develop as a result of treatment with PDT. Fever, nausea, and vomiting have been reported infrequently. I understand that I will be closely monitored for adverse effects, allergic reactions, and changes in laboratory test results and will be treated for any that might arise.

The safety of using PHOTOFRIN II during pregnancy has not been established. I understand, therefore, that if I am a woman of childbearing capability, I cannot be pregnant at the time of entering this study and that I will be practicing a medically acceptable form of birth control through the study period.

3. I understand that benefits to myself and others that may occur as a result of my participation in this study are: demonstration of whether the use of photodynamic therapy (PHOTOFRIN II plus light) following surgical removal of urinary bladder tumors will retard or eliminate the return of cancerous tissue as compared with surgery alone; close observation to determine my progress, and rapid response to possible recurrence of my disease.

4. Alternative treatments for my condition may include: immunotherapy, regional infusion chemotherapy, and combined therapy and chemotherapy. I understand that my doctor will discuss the advantages and disadvantages of these treatments with me.

5. I understand that information arising as the result of my participation in this study will be handled in a confidential manner. I also understand that representatives of QLT Phototherapeutics, Inc., (American Cyanamid Company/

Lederle Laboratories)—who is sponsoring the studies of PHOTOFRIN II—and/or the Food and Drug Administration (FDA) may review my records; however, they are obliged by law to keep the information confidential. If the results of this study are ever reported publicly or published, I understand that my name will not be disclosed.

6. I understand that in the event of physical injury or physical illness resulting from this research procedure, no monetary compensation will be made but any immediate emergency medical treatment that may be necessary will be made available to me without charge. Further information may be obtained from:

Name of Physician—Principal Investigator

Hospital Name   Street Address

City   State   Zip   Telephone Number

7. I understand that I may contact _____
M.D., Principal Investigator at _____
Hospital, located at _____
(Telephone: _____) if I have any questions regarding injury related to the research.

8. I certify that I have read the preceding or that it has been read to me and that I understand its contents, and that I have discussed the above facts with my physician and have been given the opportunity to ask questions, which have been answered to my satisfaction. Any questions I have pertaining to the research have been or will be answered by Dr. _____. A copy of this consent form will be given to me. I understand that my participation in the study is voluntary and that neither my refusal to participate nor my discontinuing participation will involve penalty or loss of benefits to which I am otherwise entitled.

My signature below means that I have freely agreed to participate in this experimental study.

Date   Signature

(Courtesy of Western Institute for Laser Treatment.)

INDEX